The #1 Cookbook

Over 170+ of the MOST Popular Recipes Across 7 Different Cuisines!

(Breakfast, Lunch & Dinner)

by Olivia Rogers

Copyright © 2017 By Olivia Rogers
All rights reserved. No part of this book may be reproduced in any form without permission in writing from the author. No part of this publication may be reproduced or transmitted in any form or by any means, mechanic, electronic, photocopying, recording, by any storage or retrieval system, or transmitted by email without the permission in writing from the author and publisher.
For information regarding permissions write to author at
Olivia@TheMenuAtHome.com
Reviewers may quote brief passages in review.

Please note that credit for the images used in this book go to the respective owners.
You can view this at: TheMenuAtHome.com/image-list

Olivia Rogers
TheMenuAtHome.com

Table of Contents

Introduction — 10
1. Egg & Salmon Sandwich — 10
2. Creamy Blueberry-Pecan Oatmeal — 11
3. Mexi-Melt — 12
4. Tutti-Frutti Muesli — 12
5. Breakfast Mini Pizza — 13
6. Thermos-Ready Smoothie — 14
7. Rhuarb Fruit Salad — 15
8. Breakfast Parfait — 16
9. Pineapple-Raspberry Parfaits — 16
10. Purple Fruit Smoothie — 17
11. Pumpkin Oatmeal — 18
12. Banana Tortilla Sandwich/Burrito — 19
13. Overnight Oatmeal — 20
14. Poached Eggs — 20
15. Florentine Hash Skillet — 21
16. Cranberry Muesli — 22
17. Bagel Gone Bananas — 23
18. Crunchy Granola Wedges — 24
19. Green Smoothie — 25
20. Chocolate Banana Oatmeal — 26
21. Coconut Chai-Spiced Oatmeal — 27
22. Blueberries with Lemon Cream — 28
23. Fig & Ricotta Oatmeal — 28
24. New York Sunday Breakfast — 29

25. Savory Curry Cashew Oatmeal _____ 30
26. Date & Pine Nut Oatmeal _____ 31
27. Creamy Cherry-Walnut Oatmeal _____ 32
28. Quick Breakfast Taco _____ 33
29. Crunchy Cerebral Trail Mix _____ 34
30. Yankee Grits _____ 35
31. Cherry Cream Cheese _____ 36
32. Wake-Up Smoothie _____ 37
33. Apple Oatmeal _____ 37
34. Tuna Casserole _____ 39
35. Angel Hair Pasta Herbs French Bread Pesto Chicken _____ 40
36. Garlic Green Beans Mashed Potatoes with Chili Coke _____ 41
37. Garlic Green Beans _____ 41
38. Bacon and Cheese Quiche Home Fried Potatoes _____ 42
39. Honey Pecan Pork Chops Buttered Broccoli Baked Sweet Potatoes _____ 43
40. Chicken Stroganoff Bread Tossed Salad _____ 44
41. Bubble Pizza _____ 45
42. Onion Roasted Potatoes _____ 46
43. Mexican Chicken White Rice Tortilla Chips _____ 47
44. Crock Pot Burgundy Beef Egg Noodles _____ 47
45. Down Home Baked Beans _____ 48
46. Butter Chicken _____ 49
47. Mom's Great Green Beans _____ 50
48. Chili Dogs Potato Salad _____ 51
49. Pork Tenderloin Crispy Country Baked Beans _____ 52
50. Country Baked Beans _____ 53

51. Cranberry Beef Buttered Corn Roast Baked Potatoes _____ 54
52. Baked Beans with Ham Cornbread _____ 55
53. Cornbread _____ 56
54. French Fries Cole Slaw Barbecued Beef Sandwiches _____ 57
55. KFC Coleslaw Recipe _____ 58
56. Perfect Mashed Potatoes _____ 59
57. Biscuit Pizza Casserole _____ 60
58. Blue Ribbon Chili Buttered Cornbread _____ 61
59. Vodka and Penne Sauce Italian Bread Tossed Salad _____ 62
60. Baked Corn _____ 63
61. Tater Tot Casserole Cornbread _____ 64
62. Mozzarella Chicken Garlic Pasta Italian Bread _____ 65
63. Slow Cooker Pot Roast _____ 66
64. Saltine Fried Chicken Potato Salad Corn on the Cob _____ 66
65. Brown Sugar Kielbasa Twice Baked Potatoes _____ 68
66. Onion Roasted Potatoes Salisbury steak Corn on the Cob __ 68
67. Rosemary Lemon Chicken _____ 69
68. Speedy Mediterranean chicken _____ 70
69. Seafood Bake _____ 71
70. Easy Chicken Lo Mein _____ 72
_____ 72
71. Apples Candied Sweet Potatoes with Pork Chops Dinner Rolls
_____ 73
72. Barbecued Baby Back Ribs _____ 74
73. Chili-rubbed Tilapia with Lemon and Asparagus _____ 75
74. Southwestern Corn and Pepper Casserole _____ 76
75. Fennel Crusted Sirloin _____ 77

76. Easy Chicken Taco Salad	78
77. Honey Pecan Pork Cutlets	79
78. Garlicky Steak	80
79. Curried Chicken Salad	81
80. Mango Quesadillas	82
81. Fancy Fig Sandwich	83
82. Low-Carb Roll-Up	84
83. Black Bean Wrap	85
84. Loaded Sweet Potato	86
85. Green Tortilla Pizza	87
86. Souper Spicy Soup	88
87. Hawaiian Wrap	89
88. Grilled Cheddar n' Apple	90
89. Lighter Chef's Salad	91
90. Open-Faced White Bean Sandwich	92
91. Roast Beef Roll	93
92. Niçoise Sandwich	94
93. Mediterranean Pita	96
94. Taco Salad	97
95. Quinoa Salad	98
96. Honey Soy Salmon	99
97. Spicy Veggies	99
98. Springtime Stir-Fry	100
99. Spicy Shrimp Stir-Fry	102
100. Turkey Frittata	103
101. Grilled Shrilled Skewers Over White Bean Salad	104
102. Classic Hamburger	105

103. Green Chili Bison Burger _____ 106
104. Grilled Fish Tacos _____ 107
105. Grilled Chicken with A Touch of Chili and Lime _____ 109
106. Steak, Potato Kebabs and Cilantro Sauce _____ 110
107. Moroccan Shrimp with Spinach _____ 111
108. Grilled Steak Served with Fresh Corn Salad _____ 113
109. Smoky Ham and Corn Salad _____ 114
110. Grilled Steak with Pepper Relish _____ 115
111. Mojito-Rubbed Chicken with Grilled Pineapple _____ 116
112. Spiced Pork Tenderloins with Mango Salsa _____ 118
113. Steak Sandwich with Grilled Onion _____ 119
114. Juicy Rosemary Chicken Skewer Kabobs _____ 121
115. Grilled Garlic and Pepper Steak with A Caprese Salad __ 122
116. Quick and Easy Italian Grilled Chicken _____ 124
117. Paprika Shrimp with Lemon Aioli _____ 125
118. Chicken Souvlaki with a delicious Tzatziki Sauce _____ 126
119. Sweet and Spicy Grilled Pork Tenderloin _____ 127
120. Bacon Stuffed Zucchini Boats _____ 129
121. Rosemary Stuffed, Bacon Wrapped Chicken _____ 130
122. Sweet n Spicy Grilled Pineapple Rings _____ 131
123. Hamburgers Topped with Mushrooms and Swiss Cheese _ 132
124. Tandoori Chicken Thighs _____ 133
125. Honey Flavored Grilled Shrimp _____ 134
126. Spicy Asian Pork Skewers _____ 135
127. Sweet and Savory Salmon on The Grill _____ 137
128. Delicious Black Bean Patties _____ 138
129. Honey Chicken and Vegetable Skewers _____ 139

130. Chicken Tikka Masala _____ 140
131. Tangy Grilled Chicken _____ 141
132. Stuffed Jalapenos Wrapped in Bacon _____ 143
133. Grilled Garlic and Pepper Shrimp _____ 143
134. Honey Garlic Steaks _____ 145
135. Butter Basil Shrimp _____ 146
136. London Broil _____ 147
137. Grilled Fish Tacos with A Zesty Lemon Dressing _____ 148
138. Butter Beer Chicken _____ 150
139. Fiery Shrimp _____ 152
140. Bacon Wrapped Hamburgers _____ 153
141. Grilled Zesty Tilapia with A Sweet and Spicy Mango Salsa _____ 154
142. Orange and Garlic Grilled Tuna _____ 155
143. Pineapple Chicken Tenders _____ 156
144. Pork Teriyaki Don _____ 157
145. Healthy Beef Broccoli Stir Fry _____ 158
146. Tenderloin Strips with Lemongrass _____ 160
147. Beef Stir Fry with Long Beans & Aromatic Paste _____ 161
148. Stir-fried Veggie Egg Noodles with Pork _____ 163
149. Stir-fried Vegetables Chinese Style _____ 164
150. Stir Fried Vermicelli with Chicken Teriyaki _____ 166
151. Shrimp Chili Stir Fry _____ 167
152. Chicken Rice Indian Style _____ 169
153. Quick Stir-Fried Water Spinach with Pork Rind _____ 170
154. Brown Rice with Stir-Fried Beef Teriyaki _____ 171
155. Two Sauce Pork Tenders Stir Fry _____ 172

156. Bell Pepper and Squid Stir Fry _____ 174
157. Thai-style Prawn Salad _____ 175
158. Fried Rice Oriental _____ 176
159. Pickled Eggs _____ 178
160. Tarragon Egg Salad _____ 179
161. Egg-mushroom Salad _____ 180
162. Scalloped Eggs _____ 181
163. Biscuit Sandwich _____ 182
164. Migas _____ 183
165. Greek Family Omelet _____ 184
166. The Tri-Country Special _____ 185
167. Eggs in Purgatory _____ 186
168. Moroccan Eggs _____ 187
169. Nicoise Deviled Eggs _____ 188
170. Ham Frittata _____ 189
171. Swiss Chard and Cheddar Quiche _____ 190
172. Friseé with Bacon and Soft Cooked Eggs _____ 191
173. Egg Pizza _____ 192
174. Deconstructed Croque Madame _____ 194
Conclusion _____ 196
Final Words _____ 196
Disclaimer _____ 197

Introduction

Putting together a fabulous yet simple and healthy meal should not feel like swimming upstream. This cookbook is a collection of the most delicious and tasty recipes. If you are not already on the health train, it's time to get aboard with this book's healthy recipes that taste great and are easy to make!

From day one through to the end of the month, this cookbook gives you a recipe to power your day and your health. From Egg & Salmon sandwich through to Turkey Frittata, you're going to love each and every meal presented in this book. Take your time and explore the 100+ top-rated quick and easy recipes for breakfast, lunch and dinner!

1. Egg & Salmon Sandwich

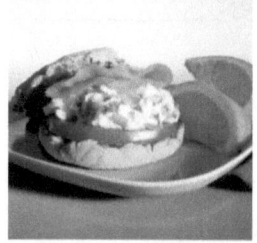

Egg whites and smoked salmon on a toasted whole-wheat muffin is a very powerful meal for breakfast.

Ingredients

- 1 tablespoon nicely chopped red onion
- Pinch of salt
- 1/2 teaspoon capers, chopped and rinsed (optional)
- 2 large egg whites, beaten
- ounce smoked salmon
- 1 slice tomato
- 1 whole-wheat English muffin, split and toasted
- 1/2 teaspoon extra-virgin olive oil

Method

1. Heat oil over medium heat. Add onion and cook. Stir to soften. Add salt, egg whites and capers. Stir for 30 seconds. For sandwich, layer smoked salmon, tomato and smoked salmon on English muffin.

Tips/Notes

For a more substantial meal, pair it with a piece of fruit or a glass of 100% juice.

2. Creamy Blueberry-Pecan Oatmeal

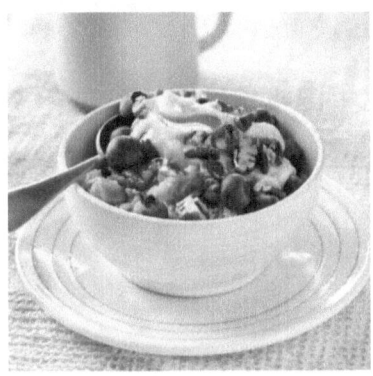

Crunchy pecans, sweet berries and protein rich Greek yogurt combine to make this healthy breakfast.

Ingredients

- 2 teaspoons pure maple syrup
- 1/2 cup old-fashioned rolled oats
- 1 cup water
- Pinch of salt
- 1/2 cup blueberries, fresh or frozen, thawed
- 1 tablespoon toasted chopped pecans
- 2 tablespoons nonfat plain Greek yogurt

Method

1. Boil water and salt in a saucepan. Stir in oats. Cook at medium heat and stir about 5 minutes. Remove from heat and let it stand for 2 minutes. Top with pecans, syrup, yogurt and blueberries.

Tips/Notes

Blueberries help lower the amount of cholesterol in blood, reducing the risk of heart-related diseases.

3. Mexi-Melt

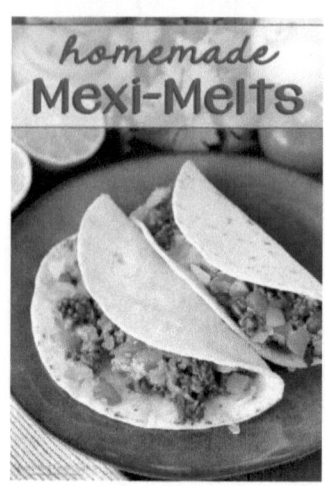

Spread refried beans on whole-wheat toast. Top with cheese and salsa for a powerful breakfast.

Ingredients

- 1 tablespoon shredded cheese, e.g. Jack or Mexican blend
- 1 slice toasted, whole-wheat bread
- 1 tablespoon prepared salsa
- 2 tablespoons canned nonfat refried beans

Method

1. Spread refried beans on whole-wheat toast. Top with salsa and cheese. Microwave on high heat to melt cheese.

Tips/Notes

Salsa is low in calories, has no fats and is rich in Lycopenes—a great antioxidant that's characteristic of tomatoes.

4. Tutti-Frutti Muesli

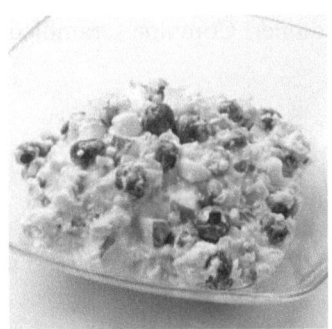

Yogurt mixed with fruit packs and muesli satisfies all morning long.

Ingredients

- 1/2 cup low-fat or non-fat plain yogurt
- 1-2 teaspoons pure maple syrup or honey
- 1/4 cup unsweetened muesli
- 1/4 cup diced banana
- 1/4 cup diced apple
- 1/2 cup blueberries, frozen or fresh (thawed)

Method

1. Stir together blueberries, yogurt, muesli, banana and apple. Add maple syrup or honey to taste.

Tips/Notes

Adding a banana to your diet helps keep the bowels healthy and provides nutrients that regulate heart rhythm.

5. Breakfast Mini Pizza

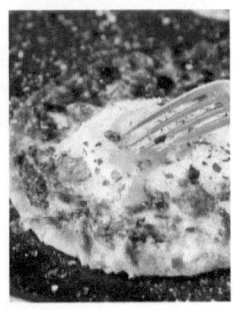

Pizza is not just made for dinner! Combine scrambled eggs and mini pizzas for a breakfast you'll love.

Ingredients

- 1 large egg, beaten
- 2 tablespoons shredded Italian cheese blend
- 1 whole-wheat English muffin, (toasted and split)
- 2 slices pepperoni
- 2 tablespoons prepared marinara sauce

Method

1. Pre-heat toaster oven boiler. Coat a nonstick skillet with cooking spray. Heat over medium heat. Add egg, cook and stir for 1 minute. Spread marina sauce on English muffin halves. Top with cheese, pepperoni and scrambled egg. Boil for 2 minutes to melt cheese.

Tips/Notes

Unlike what most people know about pepperoni, this ingredient *contains complete proteins, minerals and B vitamins.*

6. Thermos-Ready Smoothie

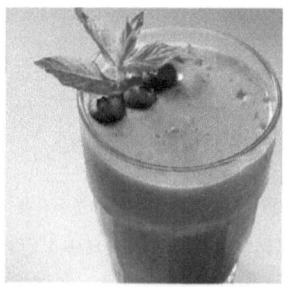

This breakfast meal is protein and fiber-rich to power your morning.

Ingredients

- 1/2 banana
- 1/4 cup silken tofu
- 1/2 cup apple juice
- 1 cup frozen mixed berries

Method

1. Combine tofu, banana, apple juice and berries in a blender. Blend to smooth.

Tips/Notes

Apple juice contains disease fighting vitamins and powerful phytonutrients which counter asthma and cancer.

7. Rhuarb Fruit Salad

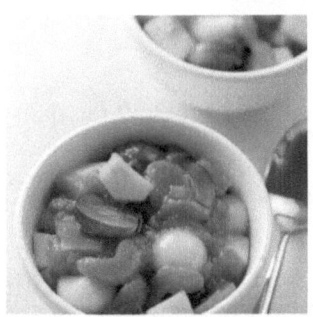

Rhubarb meets orange liqueur and a little honey for a tangy "sauce" to toss with melon, strawberries, grapes and mango.

Ingredients

- 1 1/2 cups sliced green or red grapes
- 2 tablespoons Cointreau or Grand Marnier
- 1 1/2 cups cantaloupe balls, small honeydew or pieces
- 3 tablespoons honey
- 1 1/2 cups sliced strawberries or mango
- 3 cups thinly sliced fresh rhubarb

Method

1. Stir grapes, melon and strawberries (or mango) into the rhubarb mixture. Serve or return to the refrigerator to chill further.

2. Bring Conintreau (Grand Marnier), honey and rhubarb to simmer in medium heat. Cook, stir for 4 minutes. Transfer to a bigger bowl and refrigerate for 10 minutes

Tips/Notes

Mangoes are without doubt the most consumed fruit in the world. They are a low calorie, low fat and cholesterol-free source of an endless list of nutrients.

8. Breakfast Parfait

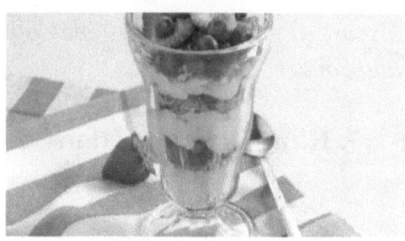

Some vitamin-rich fruit and a little low-fat dairy to kick start your day, nutritionally speaking.

Ingredients

- 1 cup papaya chunks, pineapple chunks or cling peaches
- 2 teaspoons toasted wheat germ
- 3/4 cup low-fat cottage cheese or low-fat plain yogurt

Method

1. Place yogurt or cottage cheese in a bowl. Sprinkle with wheat germ. Top with fruit.

Tips/Notes

Papaya is one of those fruits that the body needs for a healthy *immune system.*

9. Pineapple-Raspberry Parfaits

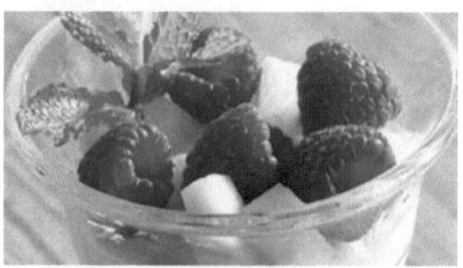

Spark your morning by serving dessert after assembling these quick parfaits.

Ingredients

- (2 cups) nonfat peach yogurt
- 1 1/2 cups frozen, canned or fresh pineapple chunks
- 1 1/2 cups pint fresh raspberries

Method

1. Divide and layer raspberries, pineapple and yogurt into 4 glasses. Serve.

Tips/Notes

Peach yogurt contains calcium and vitamin D necessary for the proper functioning of the skeletal system.

10. Purple Fruit Smoothie

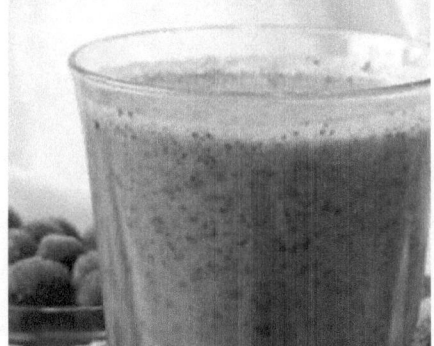

This meal is fully packed with vitamins; a perfect way to get your body and mind ready for the long day ahead.

Ingredients

- 2 Frozen Bananas (skins peeled)
- 1/2 Cup of Frozen Blueberries
- 1 Cup of Juice preferably orange

Optional

- 1 Tablespoon of Vanilla extract or Honey (to add Sweetness and Consistency to Blended Treat)
- Protein Powder of your choice to add a little bit of oomph and power your morning.

Method

1. Place all ingredients in a blender (use more or less juice to vary the thickness of the smoothie). Blend for 2 minutes. Enjoy!

Tips/Notes

Orange juice contains high levels of vitamin C which means health benefits *for your heart, skin and weight.*

11. Pumpkin Oatmeal

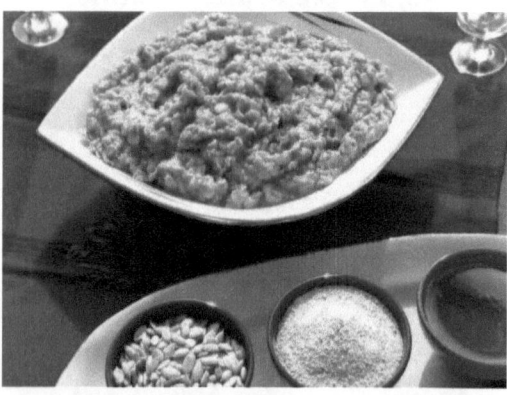

Begin your day with a great burst of flavor, vitamins and whole grains. Stay full through to lunch.

Ingredients

- 1/2 Cup of Canned Pumpkin Puree
- 3/4 Cup Milk
- 1 Cup of Quick Cooking rolled oats (Switch it up with cream wheat or other oats such as steel cut oats)
- 1/4 Teaspoon of Pumpkin Pie Spice
- 1 Teaspoon of Cinnamon Sugar

Method

1. Mix milk and oats together in a microwave-safe bowl for 2 minutes. Stir the oats. Add more milk (if you want to vary the density). Microwave again for 45 seconds. Stir in the pumpkin pie spice, pumpkin puree and cinnamon sugar. Serve when cool.

Tips/Notes

Have a healthier heart with pumpkin oatmeal recipe!

12. Banana Tortilla Sandwich/Burrito

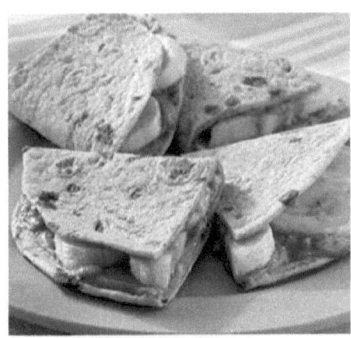

This is a simple twist on an American Staple and is a favorite of many!

Ingredients

- 1 (6 Inch) Flour Tortilla
- Honey
- Peanut Butter, Hazelnut or Almond Butter to switch it up
- Raisins
- Banana

Method

1. Spread peanut butter on tortilla. Drizzle honey and raisins to add flavor. Place a peeled banana on the tortilla. Wrap and enjoy!

Tips/Notes

Raisins are among the best concentrated sources of numerous health-benefiting electrolytes, polyphenolic antioxidants, dietary fiber, and vitamins.

13. Overnight Oatmeal

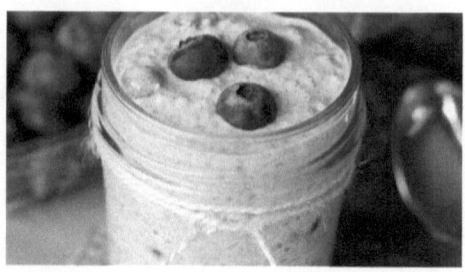

Here is a great meal to keep you full and going throughout your morning.

Ingredients

- 1/3 cup dried cranberries
- 2 cups steel-cut oats
- 1/3 cup dried chopped apricots
- 1/8 teaspoon salt to taste
- 4 cups water

Method

1. Mix water, dried cranberries, oats, dried apricots and salt in a 5/6-quart slow cooker. Turn the heat to low. Cover with lid and cook.

Tips/Notes

Apricots have numerous health benefits including the ability to treat constipation, earache, skin diseases, fevers, anemia, cancer and indigestion.

14. Poached Eggs

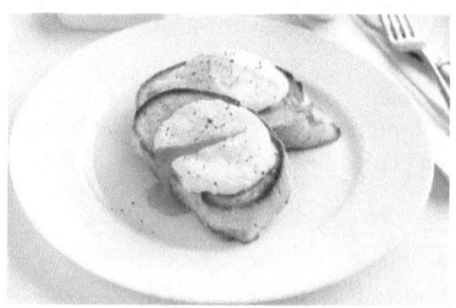

There are several ways to poach an egg. We tried them all and this was the winning method!

Ingredients

- 1/4 cup distilled white vinegar
- 4 large eggs

Method

1. Break eggs into a bowl. Fill a Dutch oven or straight sided skillet with 2 inches of water and bring to boil. Add vinegar. Reduce to a gentle simmer. Submerging the lip of the bowl into the simmering water, add eggs (gently).

2. Cook for 8 minutes for hard set, 5minutes for medium set and 4 minutes for soft set. Allow the eggs to drain by using a slotted spoon to transfer the eggs to a dish towel for 1 minute.

Tips/Notes

Vinegar has shown promise in helping treat cancer, diabetes, high cholesterol and heart health.

15. Florentine Hash Skillet

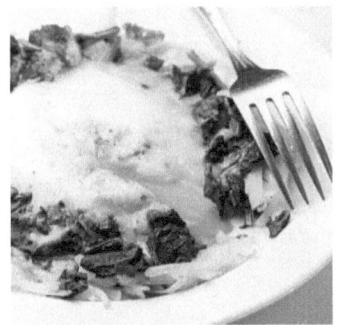

Here is a marvelous all-in-one skillet breakfast to start off your day, loaded with egg, cheese, spinach and hash browns.

Ingredients

- Pinch of freshly ground pepper
- Pinch of salt

- 2 tablespoons shredded sharp Cheddar cheese
- 1/2 cup frozen chopped spinach
- 1/2 cup precooked shredded potatoes or frozen hash browns
- 1 large egg
- 1 teaspoon extra-virgin olive oil

Method

1. Heat oil in a non-stick skillet. Turn heat to medium. Layer spinach and browns into the pan. Crack the egg on top. Sprinkle with cheese, pepper and salt. Turn heat to medium low and cover. Cook until cheese is melted, egg is set and hash browns turn brown.

Tips/Notes

Olive oil has proven to be among the leading concentrated sources of healthy fats and anti-oxidants.

16. Cranberry Muesli

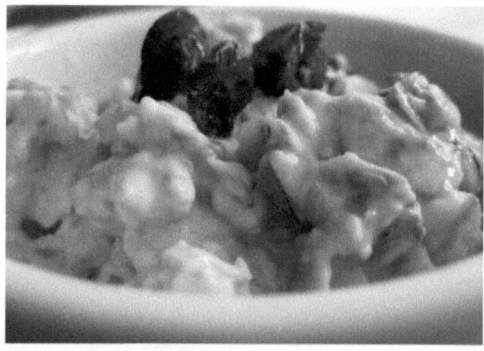

Here's a combination of nuts, yogurt, dried fruit and overnight-soaked grains. This one's modeled after the original *Wake-you-up*.

Ingredients

- 1/4 teaspoon vanilla extract
- 1 tablespoon unsalted sunflower seeds
- 2 teaspoons honey
- 2 tablespoons dried cranberries
- 1/2 cup unsweetened or fruit-juice-sweetened cranberry juice
- 1 tablespoon wheat germ
- 1/8 teaspoon salt

- 1/2 cup low-fat plain yogurt
- 6 tablespoons old-fashioned rolled oats, (not steel or quick-cooking cut)

Method

1. Combine vanilla, honey, wheat germ, sunflower seeds, cranberries, oats, juice, yogurt and salt in bowl. Cover. Refrigerate.

Tips/Notes

One of the major benefits of oats and sunflower seeds is that they are building blocks for cell membranes, allowing you your body to balance hormones.

17. Bagel Gone Bananas

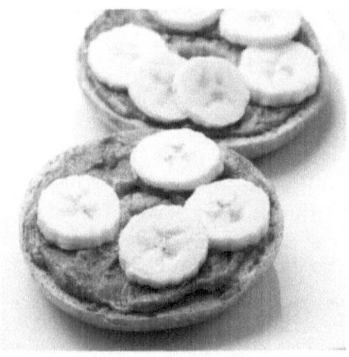

Talk about a healthy powerful breakfast: this special bagel topped with banana slices and nut butter will be ready in no time!

Ingredients

- 1 small banana, sliced
- 2 tablespoons natural nut butter, e.g. peanut, almond or cashew
- Pinch of salt
- 1 teaspoon honey
- 1 whole-wheat bagel, split and toasted

Method

1. Stir together honey, nut butter and salt in a bowl. Divide the mixture between bagel halves. Top with banana slices.

Tips/Notes

From fighting drunkenness, dandruffs to treating fevers and cuts, honey is another powerhouse of nutrients.

18. Crunchy Granola Wedges

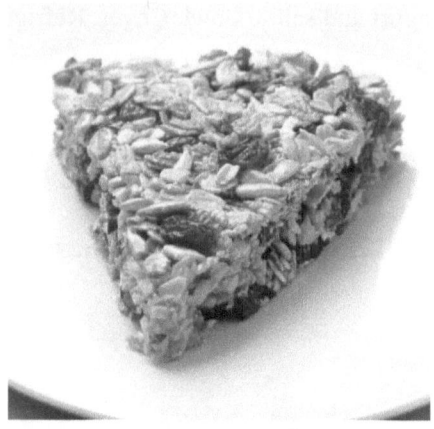

Substitute your favorite nuts and/or seeds, fruit, for sunflower seeds and/or dried cranberries in these granola bars.

Ingredients

- 1 cup chopped nuts or sunflower seeds
- 1 cup rolled oats
- 1/2 cup honey
- 1 cup wheat flakes
- Pinch of salt
- 1 cup dried cranberries

Method

1. Pre-heat oven to 400°F. Spread wheat flakes, seeds (nuts) and oats on a baking sheet. Bake to fragrant and starting to brown for about 10 minutes. Coat a pie pan with cooking spray.

2. Cook 1/2 cup honey in a saucepan over medium heat (Don't stir). Wait until edges begin to darken (4 minutes). Pour the toasted oat mixture into the honey. Add salt and cranberries. Stir until completely coated.

3. Press the granola into the pie pan using a spatula coated with cooking spray. Let it cool. Slice into wedges. Transfer it to a wire rack to cool completely.

Tips/Notes

Wheat flakes are the answer to controlling obesity. It also contains nutrients best for the brain.

19. Green Smoothie

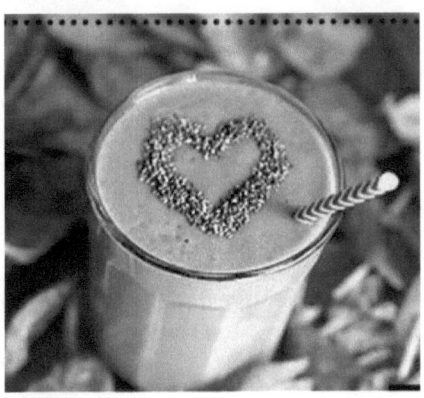

Get a dose of the dark leafy greens with this tasty green smoothie for breakfast.

Ingredients

- 2 medium-ripe bananas
- 1 tablespoon ground flaxseed
- 1 ripe apple or pear, peeled and chopped if desired
- 1/2 cup cold orange juice
- 2 cups chopped kale leaves
- 12 ice cubes
- 1/2 cup cold water

Method

1. Place flaxseed, ice cubes, orange juice, kale, bananas, water, apple (or pear) and bananas in a blender. Pulse a few times. Puree until smooth while scraping down the sides as desired.

Tips/Notes

Surprisingly, even spinach does not come close to the amount of vitamins kale provides.

20. Chocolate Banana Oatmeal

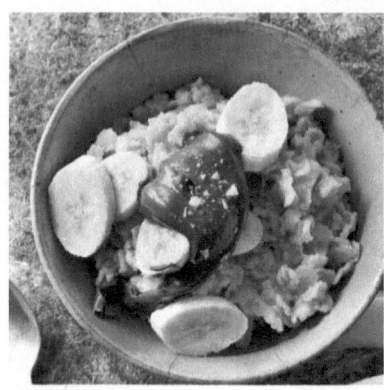

Have a little luxury with this friendly healthy banana and chocolate oatmeal recipe. You may want to try overnight variation.

Ingredients

- Pinch of salt
- 1 tablespoon chocolate-hazelnut spread
- 1/2 small banana, sliced
- Pinch of flaky sea salt
- 1/2 cup old-fashioned rolled oats

Method

1. Ring a pinch of salt and water to boil. Stir in oats and boil. Turn heat to medium and cook, stirring occasionally for about 5 minutes. Remove from fat. Cover and let it stand for 3 minutes. Top with chocolate spread, flaky salt and banana.

Tips/Notes

Also known as filberts, hazelnuts are a sweet-flavored nut that can be added to snacks, baked recipes.

21. Coconut Chai-Spiced Oatmeal

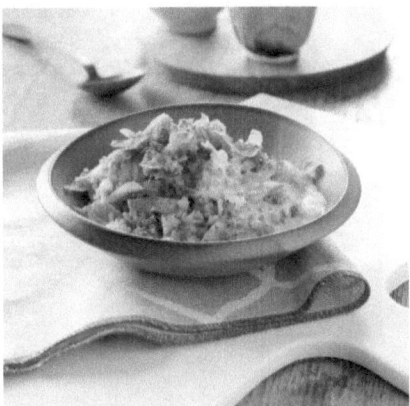

This powerful recipe is a great upgrade from the plain cinnamon and brings with it the flavors of coconut and chai tea.

Ingredients

- 1/8 teaspoon ground ginger
- 2 teaspoons brown sugar
- 1 cup water
- Pinch of ground pepper
- Pinch of ground cardamom
- 1/4 teaspoon ground cinnamon
- 2 tablespoons toasted unsweetened coconut chips
- 3 tablespoons unsweetened coconut milk beverage
- 1/2 cup old-fashioned rolled oats
- Pinch of salt, divided

Method

1. Bring salt and water to boil. Stir in oats and reduce heat to medium. Cook and stir occasionally for 5 minutes. Remove from heat. Cover and let it stand for 3 minutes. Top with coconut chips, coconut beverage, cinnamon, cardamom, pepper, ginger and brown sugar.

Tips/Notes

Cinnamon has a plethora or health benefits but the major one is its ability to reduce heart disease risk factors. It also helps reduce blood sugar levels.

22. Blueberries with Lemon Cream

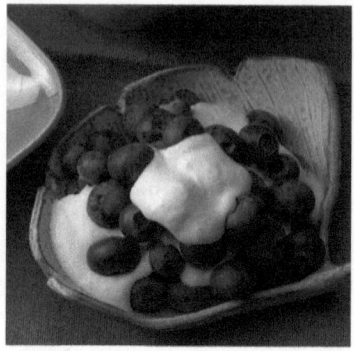

Blending reduced-fat-cream cheese and vanilla yogurt creates a virtuous and delicious topping. You may use any fresh berry in this recipe.

Ingredients

- 4 ounces reduced-fat cream cheese, (Neufchatel)
- 2 cups fresh blueberries
- 2 teaspoons freshly grated lemon zest
- 1 teaspoon honey
- 3/4 cup low-fat vanilla yogurt

Method

1. Break up cream cheese using a fork. Drain any liquid from the yogurt. Add yogurt and honey Use an electric mixer. Beat at high speed to a creamy mixture. Stir in lemon zest. Layer blueberries and lemon cream in wineglass or dessert dishes and enjoy!

Tips/Notes

Lemon zest helps ward off and treat cancer. Also, they are very powerful health rejuvenators in eradicating toxic elements in the body.

23. Fig & Ricotta Oatmeal

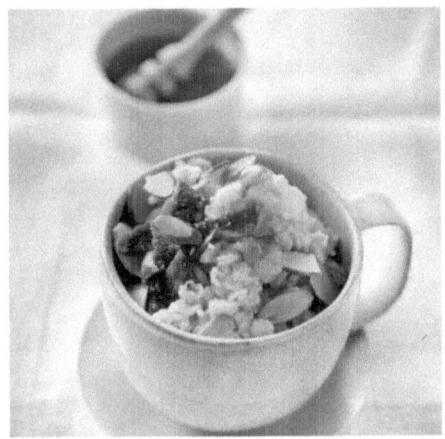

Creamy ricotta, crunchy almonds and sweet figs make this a very healthy breakfast meal.

Ingredients

- Pinch of salt
- 1/2 cup old-fashioned rolled oats
- 2 tablespoons part-skim ricotta cheese
- 1 cup water
- 2 teaspoons honey
- 2 tablespoons chopped dried figs
- 1 tablespoon toasted sliced almonds

Method

1. Bring salt and water to boil. Stir in oats. Turn heat to medium heat and cook. Stir occasionally for about 5 minutes. Remove from heat. Top with figs, almonds, ricotta and honey.

Tips/Notes

Figs have numerous health benefits which include its use in the treatment of sexual dysfunction, indigestion, diabetes, bronchitis, cough, asthma, piles and constipation.

24. New York Sunday Breakfast

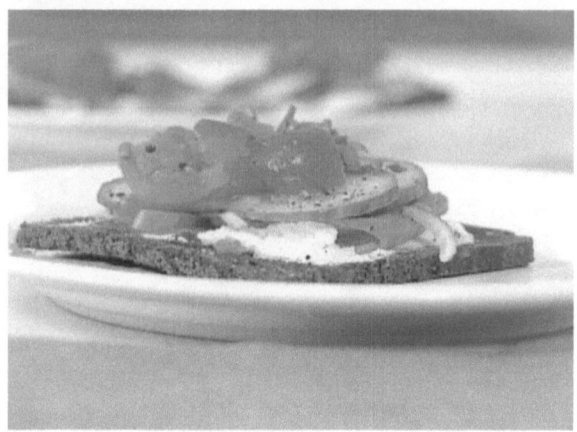

Here's an updated version of a very popular breakfast, lox and bagels.

Ingredients

- 8 pieces packaged, thin pumpernickel bread
- 1/4 cup whipped cream cheese
- 1/2 red onion, thinly sliced
- 8 ounces thinly sliced smoked salmon
- 2 teaspoons fresh, chopped chives
- Pepper and salt
- 2 medium tomatoes, seeded, core, and diced
- 1/4 English cucumber, thinly sliced

Method

1. Toast the bread. Spread cream cheese on top of each piece. Put a couple of onion slices, smoked salmon, chopped tomato and slices of cucumber on top. Season with pepper and salt and sprinkle with chives.

Tips/Notes

The spring garden turns very attractive when the chives bloom in May and June. It's not just about beauty, they also help fight hypertension, minimize the risk of getting cancer, particularly prostate cancer.

25. Savory Curry Cashew Oatmeal

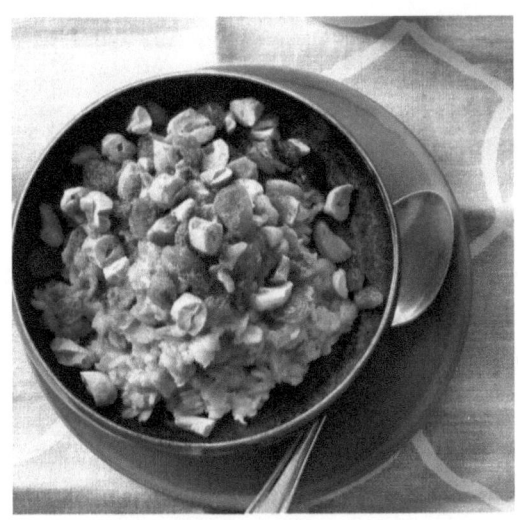

Spruce up your morning routine with this savory recipe with curry powder, raisins and curry. If you require more sweetness, sprinkle a little honey on top.

Ingredients

- 1 cup water
- 1/2 cup old-fashioned rolled oats
- Pinch of salt
- 1/4 teaspoon curry powder
- 2 tablespoons toasted chopped cashews
- 3 tablespoons golden raisins

Method

1. Bring salt and water to boil. Stir in oats. Bring heat to medium and cook. Stir occasionally for 5 minutes. Remove from heat and cover. Let it cool before adding cashews, curry powder and raisins.

Tips/Notes

Cashews are packed with antioxidants, minerals and are full of energy for robust health.

26. Date & Pine Nut Oatmeal

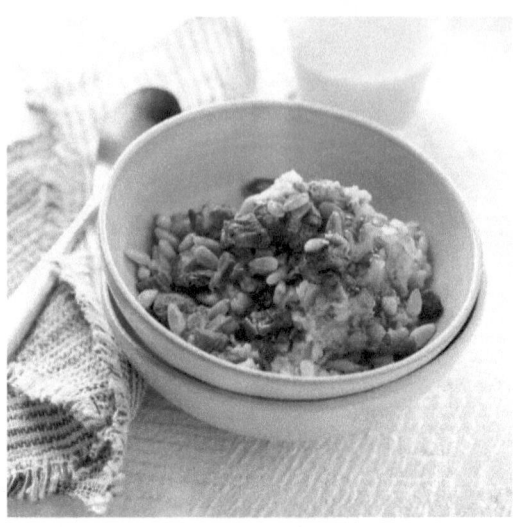

This recipe comes with sweet dried dates, honey, cinnamon and pine nuts for the best breakfast flavor.

Ingredients

- 1/4 teaspoon ground cinnamon
- 1 teaspoon honey
- Pinch of salt
- 1/2 cup old-fashioned rolled oats
- 1 cup water
- 2 tablespoons chopped dates
- 1 tablespoon toasted pine nuts

Method

1. Bring salt and water to boil. Stir in oats. Turn heat to medium. Cook and stir. Remove from heat before topping with pine nuts, cinnamon, honey and dates.

Tips/Notes

Dates are a great source of health benefits for the brain, colon and heart.

27. Creamy Cherry-Walnut Oatmeal

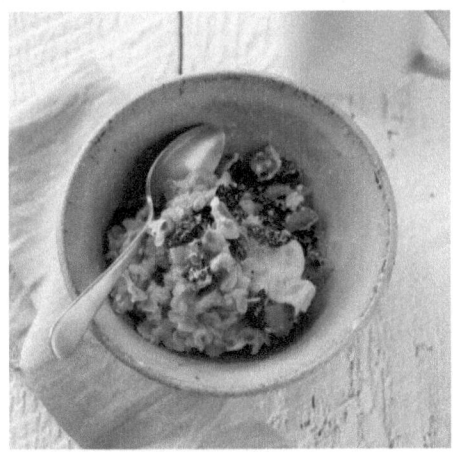

Dried cherries, lemon zest and cream cheese, gives this recipe a cheesecake-like flavor.

Ingredients

- 1 tablespoon chopped dried cherries
- 1 cup water
- 2 teaspoons raw cane sugar, such as turbinado
- Pinch of salt
- 1 tablespoon toasted chopped walnuts
- 1/2 teaspoon lemon zest
- 1/2 cup old-fashioned rolled oats
- 1 tablespoon reduced-fat cream cheese

Method

1. Bring salt and water to boil. Stir in oats. Turn heat to medium. Cook and stir. Remove from heat before topping with cherries, lemon zest, sugar, walnuts and cream cheese.

Tips/Notes

Clinical research and nutritional facts report that walnuts contain omega 3s, aids in weight management and heart health.

28. Quick Breakfast Taco

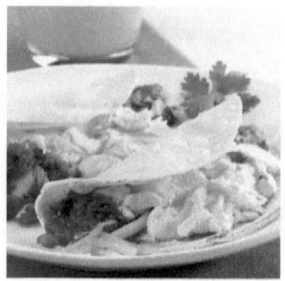

This is cousin of the popular burrito breakfast meal with egg substitute and reduced-fat cheddar.

Ingredients

- 1 tablespoon salsa
- 2 corn tortillas
- 1/2 cup liquid egg substitute, e.g. Egg beaters
- 2 tablespoons shredded reduced-fat Cheddar cheese

Method

1. Top tortillas with cheese and salsa. Heat to melt cheese. Coat a small non-skillet with cooking spray. Turn heat to medium. Add egg substitute. Cook, stirring occasionally (about 1.5 minutes). Divide scrambled egg between the tacos.

Tips/Notes

Taco recipes turn up the heat but keep the calorie count as low as possible.

29. Crunchy Cerebral Trail Mix

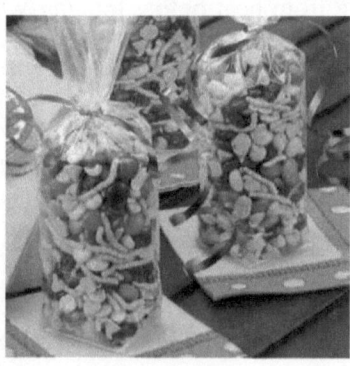

Crunchy, sweet and salty, this simple trail mix combines all your favorite flavors in a convenient mix.

Ingredients

- 2 teaspoons raisins
- 1/4 cup Cheerios
- 2 teaspoons semi-sweet mini chocolate chips
- 1 tablespoon pepitas

Method

1. Combine pepitas, cheerios, chocolate chips and raisins in a small bowl. Serve.

Tips/Notes

Clinical research studies show that cheerios help reduce and manage bad cholesterol levels.

30. Yankee Grits

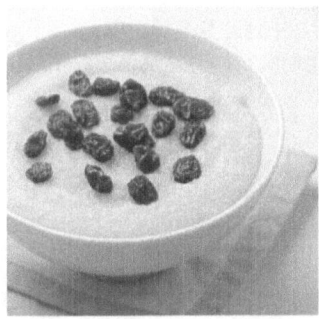

Milk and sweet maple syrup give this satisfying recipe the staying power.

Ingredients

- 1 cup water or low-fat milk
- Pinch of salt
- 2 teaspoons pure maple syrup
- 2 tablespoons chopped dried fruit, raisins or dried cranberries
- 1/4 cup quick-cooking grits

Method

1. Bring water or milk, salt and syrup to boil. Turn heat to high. Whisk in grits slowly. Turn heat to medium low. Cover and cook, stirring occasionally for about 4 minutes. Sprinkle with dried fruit

Tips/Notes

Low fat milk helps reduce calories and obesity. It doesn't go without mentioning that it's also best consumed during pregnancy.

31. Cherry Cream Cheese

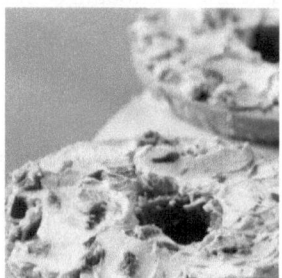

We all like the flavor of cherries. Spread them on your morning sandwich or bagel between crackers for that cherry-inspired snack

Ingredients

- 1 1/2 teaspoons confectioners' sugar
- 4 ounces non-fat cream cheese
- Pinch of ground allspice
- 1/4 cup thawed and drained frozen cherries or chopped pitted fresh cherries

Method

1. Combine cherries, cream cheese, allspice and sugar in a small bowl. Serve.

Tips/Notes

Experiencing insomnia, belly fat and joint pain? Here is a perfect meal you don't want to leave behind.

32. Wake-Up Smoothie

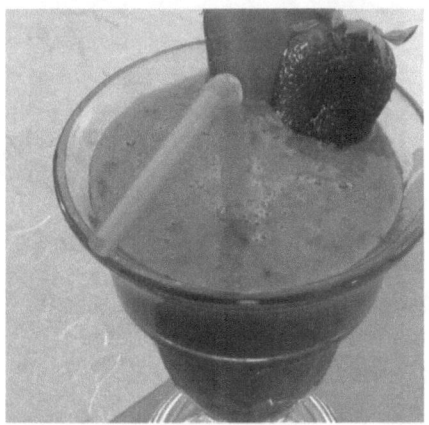

A stash of berries in your freezer can jump start your morning with its nutritious tasty smoothie.

Ingredients

- 1 1/4 cups orange juice
- 1 banana
- 1 1/4 cups berries (frozen) e.g. blackberries, raspberries, strawberries and/or blueberries
- 1/2 cup low-fat plain yogurt or low-fat silken tofu
- 1 tablespoon Splenda Granular or sugar

Method

1. Combine banana, orange juice, yogurt (tofu), berries and sugar in a blender. Cover and blend. Serve immediately.

Tips/Notes

This breakfast meal provides vitamin C, fiber, potassium and soy protein.

33. Apple Oatmeal

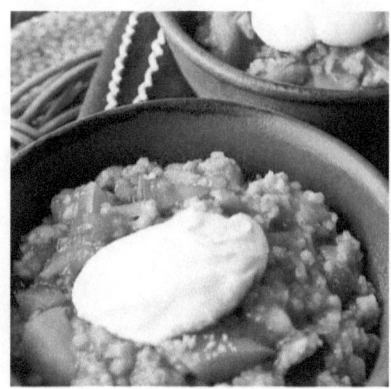

This recipe entails cook apples and oats, whole grains and a tasty fruit serving.

Ingredients

- 4 crisp apples, e.g. Pink Lady, Jazz, divided
- 3 tablespoons brown sugar, divided
- 1/4 teaspoon salt
- 1 cup steel-cut oats
- 1/2 cup nonfat plain Greek yogurt
- 4 cups water
- 1/2 teaspoon ground cinnamon

Method

1. Using a box grater, shred 2 apples. Leave the core behind. Turn heat to medium-high heat. Add oats and cook. Stir until toasted. Add the shredded apples and water. Bring to boil.

2. Turn heat to maintain simmer and cook. Stir frequently for 10 minutes. Chop the remaining 2 apples. Stir in chopped apples after oats have cooked.

3. Add 2 brown sugar, salt and cinnamon; continue cooking and stirring for about 15 minutes. Divide and top each portion of oatmeal with yogurt and 3/4 teaspoon brown sugar.

Tips/ Notes

Apple oatmeal promotes an overall healthy eating pattern. Other health benefits include weight loss, nervous health and heart function.

34. Tuna Casserole

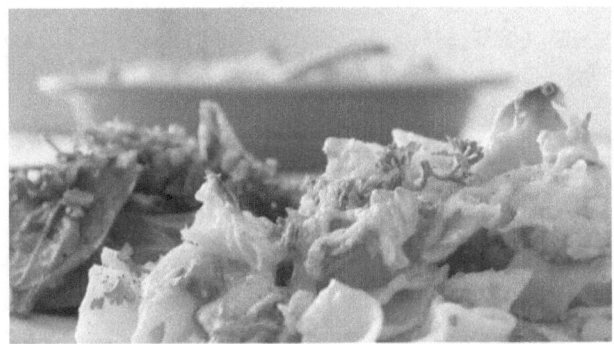

This is a comforting and reliable classic recipe that features cheese, milk, macaroni and tuna. It's an all-star, easy-to-follow recipe.

Ingredients

- 2 Tablespoons butter
- 1/4 cup grape nuts
- 1 small onion, chopped
- 1/4 cup milk
- 1/2 teaspoon dry mustard
- 1/2 teaspoon garlic
- 1 small package cream cheese
- 1 Can tuna
- 1 Can Campbell's Cream of Celery Soup
- 2 cups macaroni

Method

1. Cook macaroni according to package instructions. Mix softened cream cheese, milk and cream of celery until smooth.

2. Add garlic, onion, mustard and tuna. Stir in cooked macaroni. Mix grape in melted butter. Spread mixture over casserole. Bake in 375 degrees for 45 minutes.

Tips/Notes

When eaten in moderation, tuna brings so many benefits among them avoiding negative effects brought about high levels of mercury in food.

35. Angel Hair Pasta Herbs French Bread Pesto Chicken

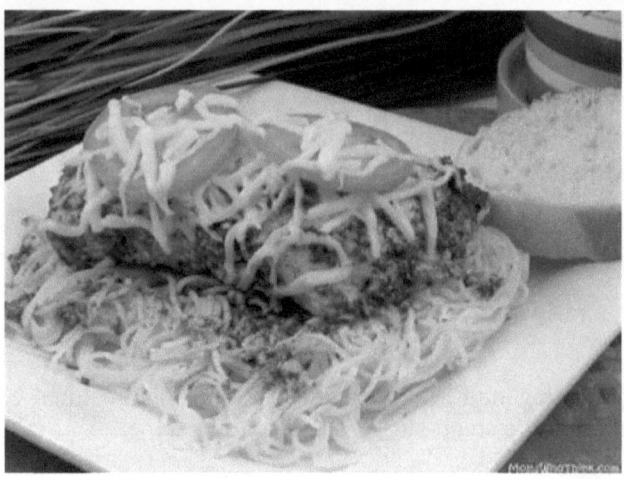

This recipe contains chicken breasts, tomato and cheese to keep you powered throughout the afternoon.

Ingredients

- Shredded mozzarella cheese
- 2 plum tomatoes
- 1/2 cup basil pesto
- 4 boneless skinless chicken breasts

Method

1. Pre-heat oven to 350-degree F. Cover cookie with foil. Put chicken and pesto in bowl. Toss until chicken is covered. Bake for 25 minutes.

2. Sprinkle with cheese and put tomato slices on top of chicken. Bake for another 5 minutes. Serve and enjoy

Tips/Notes

Cheese comes with a host of nutrients such as proteins, calcium, vitamin A and B12. This is a perfect meal for improved eye sight, reduced blood pressure and good stomach health.

36. Garlic Green Beans Mashed Potatoes with Chili Coke

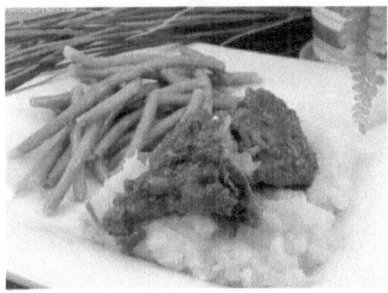

Roast mashed potatoes go perfectly well with the rest of the ingredients. It's an easy recipe!

Ingredients

- Onion soup mix
- 1 Can Cola
- 3-4 lbs. beef roast
- Chili sauce

Method

1. Cook all ingredients together until meat flakes. Serve over mashed potatoes.

Tips/Notes

Garlic could bring to an end your hair loss problems thanks to its high levels of allicin—a sulfur compound similar to that found in onions; also present in this recipe!

37. Garlic Green Beans

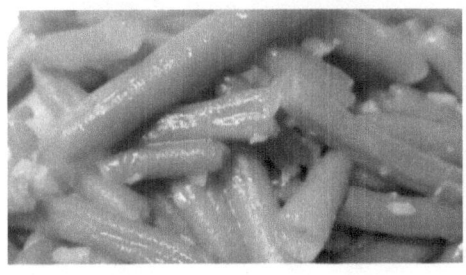

Easy and quick garlic green beans fried in garlic butter is a simple and perfect dish for garlic lovers!

Ingredients

- 2 Tablespoons butter
- 1 teaspoon garlic powder
- 2 cans regular green beans, drained

Method

1. Heat green beans. Add butter and garlic powder.

Tips/Notes

Flexible, tender green beans *are a delight of vegetarian lovers. They are a great source of dietary fiber, minerals, vitamins A and omega-3 fatty acids.*

38. Bacon and Cheese Quiche Home Fried Potatoes

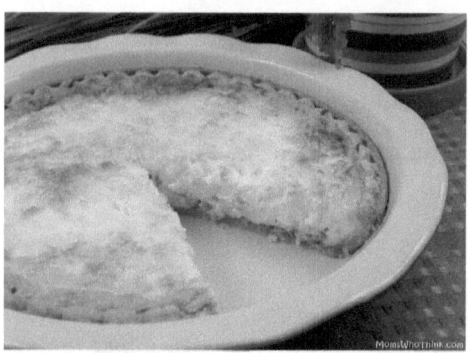

This recipe is very easy to make quiche and is also so delicious!

Ingredients

- 3/4 teaspoon salt
- 2 cup heavy cream
- 4 eggs
- 1 bag Italian blend shredded cheese (or mozzarella cheese)
- 12 bacon slices, crumbled
- 1 Tablespoon butter
- 1 9-inch pie crust, unbaked

Method

1. Preheat oven to 425 degrees F. Spread the crust into quiche or pie plate. Spread butter over crust. Sprinkle cheese and bacon on crust.

2. Beat eggs together with the remaining ingredients. Pour them into crust. Bake 20 minutes. Turn down heat to 325 degrees. Bake for 30 more min. Serve when cool

Tips/Notes

This recipe is a great source of calories from fat. It also contains dietary fibre, carbohydrates and a sufficient amount of potassium.

39. Honey Pecan Pork Chops Buttered Broccoli Baked Sweet Potatoes

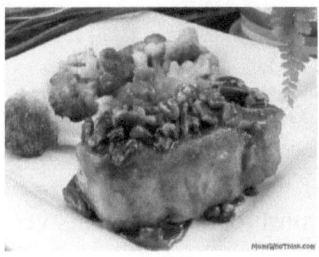

Just cook the pork cutlets in butter and you'll love this dish. Remember to serve with mashed sweet potatoes for an even greater dish!

Ingredients

- 1/4 cup chopped pecans
- 1/4 cup honey
- 2 Tablespoons butter
- Salt and pepper to taste
- 1/2 cup flour (all-purpose) for coating
- 1 1/4 pounded thin boneless pork loin

Method

1. In a small dish, mix salt, pepper and flour. Dredge the pork cutlets in flour mixture. Over medium heat, melt butter in a large skillet. Add brown, and chops both sides.

2. Transfer to a plate. Mix pecans and honey in pan drippings. Heat while stirring. Pour sauce over the cutlets. Serve with buttered broccoli and fresh baked sweet potatoes.

Tips/Notes

Unlike what most people know, sweet potatoes are a surprisingly nutritious vegetable. *Sweet potatoes possess anti-inflammatory, antioxidant and disease-fighting components.*

40. Chicken Stroganoff Bread Tossed Salad

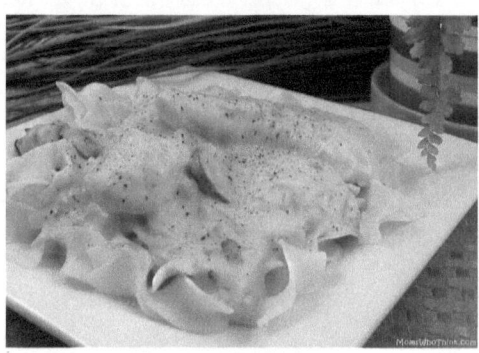

This easy recipe contains mushroom sauce. This version uses chicken in place of beef.

Ingredients

- 4 cups egg noodles
- 1/2 cup sour cream
- 1 can cream of chicken soup
- 1 medium onion, chopped
- 2 cups mushrooms
- 1 lb. chicken breast
- 2 Tablespoons butter

Method

1. Cook chicken in 1 tablespoon butter. Remove from heat. Cook onions and mushrooms in the remaining butter. Stir in sour cream and soup. Heat until boiling. Place the chicken to the pan and heat thoroughly. Serve it over tossed salad, noodles and buttered Italian bread.

Tips/Notes

This recipe contains carbohydrates, is rich in both sodium and proteins.

41. Bubble Pizza

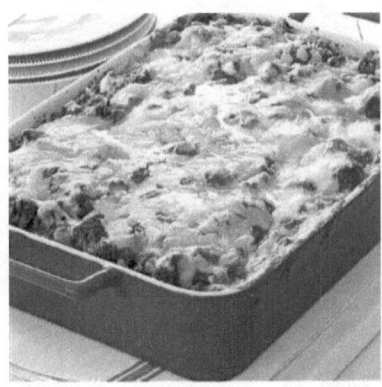

This is an easy pizza prepared with biscuit crust, cheddar mozzarella cheese and your favorite pizza toppings.

Ingredients

- 1 cup shredded cheddar cheese
- 1 1/2 cups shredded mozzarella cheese
- 2 tubes refrigerator biscuits
- 1 jar pizza sauce
- 1 1/2 lb. ground beef

Method

1. Brown beef in a large skillet drain. Mix pizza sauce and brown hamburger, mix and simmer until heated through.

2. Quarter biscuits and put them in a 13in x9in x2in greased baking bowl. Top with the beef mixture. Bake at 400 degrees F for 25 minutes. Sprinkle cheese and bake for another 10 minutes

Tips/Notes

Pizza is among the most popular options for fast food. Bubble pizza is high in sodium, calories and fat.

42. Onion Roasted Potatoes

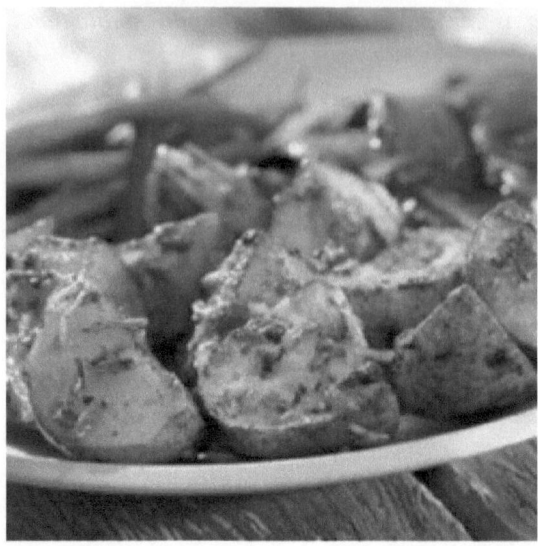

Since I learnt how to prepare onion roasted potatoes, I make them more times than I can remember.

Ingredients

- 1/3 cup olive or vegetable oil
- 2 lb. all-purpose potatoes, cut into large chunks
- 1 envelope Lipton onion recipe soup mix

Method

1. Pre-heat oven to 450 degrees F. Add all the ingredients in a large plastic bag. Put the potatoes in a shallow roasting or baking pan; discard bag.

2. Bake while stirring for 40 minutes until potatoes turn golden brown and tender. Garnish with chopped parsley (if desired). Serve potatoes and Salisbury steak with buttered corn.

Tips/Notes

Onions improve the working of vitamin C in the body therefore boosting your immunity.

43. Mexican Chicken White Rice Tortilla Chips

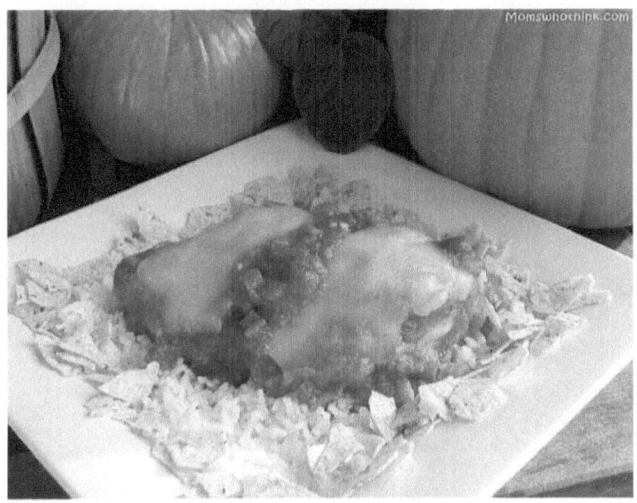

This recipe contains boneless skinless chicken, jack cheese and salsa.

Ingredients

- 1 (16 ounce) package Monterey jack cheese
- 1 jar salsa
- 4 skinless boneless chicken breasts

Method

1. Cover the chicken with salsa in a 9x13 pan. Cover with foil and bake at 350 degrees for about 20minutes and for another 25 minutes.

2. Cover chicken breast with Monterey jack cheese. Bake for 10 more minutes until cheese is melted. Serve with tortilla chips and white rice.

Tips/Notes

The health benefits of rice are endless. Rice offers instant energy, regulates and improves bowel movements and slows down the aging process.

44. Crock Pot Burgundy Beef Egg Noodles

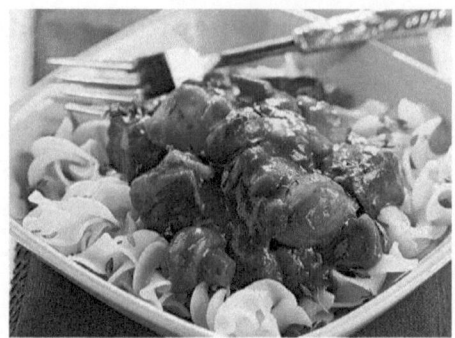

Mushrooms, the flavored sauce and tender beef served over noodles—it does get better than this!

Ingredients

- 1/4 cup burgundy wine (or cranberry juice)
- 1 Can creamy (condensed) mushroom soup
- 1 Can beefy (condensed) mushroom soup
- 2 ¼-2 ½ lbs. pot roast

Method

1. Cut meat into 1-inch pieces and trim fat. Place it a crock pot. Stir in onions, mushrooms, soup and wine (if desired). Cover and cook on high heat. Serve over cooked egg noodles.

Tips/Notes

Meat and egg noodles are a nutritional powerhouse, full of valuable nutrients such as high-quality proteins and amino acids.

45. Down Home Baked Beans

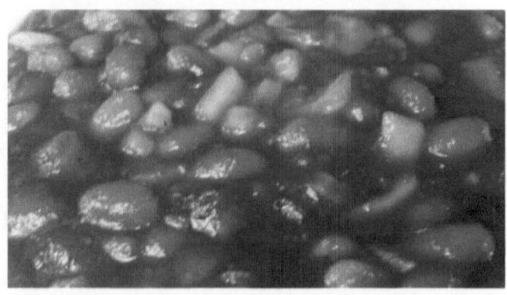

The secret ingredient in this recipe is chili sauce. This lunch dish also contains bacon, onions and brown sugar.

Ingredients

- 1-pound bacon
- 2 (28 ounce) cans baked beans
- 1 large sweet onion, chopped
- Chili sauce
- 2 cups packed brown sugar

Method

1. Pre-heat oven to 350 degrees F. Place the bacon in a big, deep skillet. Turn heat to medium heat and cook until evenly brown. Drain and crumble.

2. Combine chili sauce, bacon, brown sugar, onion and beans in a bowl. Pour the mixture into a 9x13 inch casserole dish. Bake for 40 minutes in pre-heated oven.

Tips/Notes

Home baked beans are a great source of protein. They also contain energy giving, low glycaemic index carbohydrates.

46. Butter Chicken

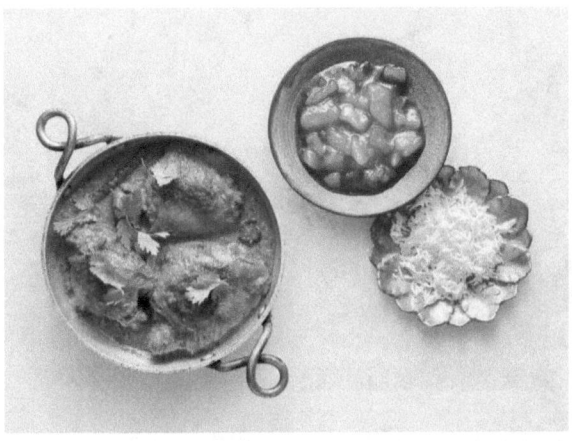

Most popular in India, the butter chicken is without doubt one of the most delicious dishes around the world.

Ingredients

- 1/2 cup butter, cut into pieces
- 4 skinless, boneless chicken breast halves
- Ground black pepper to taste
- 1/2 teaspoon garlic salt
- 1 cup buttery cracker crumbs (crushed)
- 2 eggs, beaten

Method

1. Pre-heat oven to 350 degrees F. Place cracker crumbs and eggs in two separate bowls. Mix garlic salt, pepper and cracker crumbs. Dip the chicken in eggs. Dredge in the crumb mixture to coat.

2. Place the coated chicken in a 9x13 inch dish. Place pieces of butter around the chicken. Bake for 40 minutes in a pre-heated oven.

Tips/Notes

Butter chicken is rich in protein content and supplies minerals that are very essential in losing weight and cholesterol control.

47. Mom's Great Green Beans

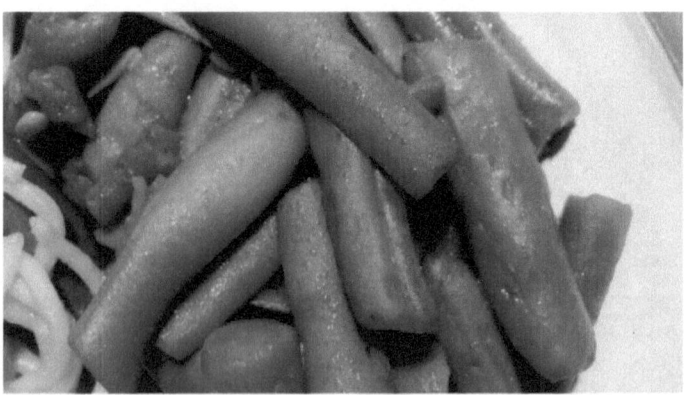

Known as Mom's Great Green Beans, this dish is easy, delicious and healthy!

Ingredients

- 1 pinch garlic pepper
- 1 beef bouillon cube
- 1 Tablespoon butter
- 1 teaspoon soy sauce
- 1 Tbsp. Worcestershire sauce
- 2 (15 ounce) cans green beans

Method

1. Drain green beans, reserving ¼ of the liquid. Immerse the bouillon cube in the liquid. Place the liquid and green beans in a saucepan. Add soy sauce, garlic pepper, Worcestershire sauce and butter to taste.

2. Light simmer for 10 minutes. Remove it from heat, leaving beans sitting in the liquid. Serve using a slotted spoon.

Tips/Notes

Looking for a dairy free and gluten-free dish for lunch? Try the Mom's Great Green Beans recipe.

48. Chili Dogs Potato Salad

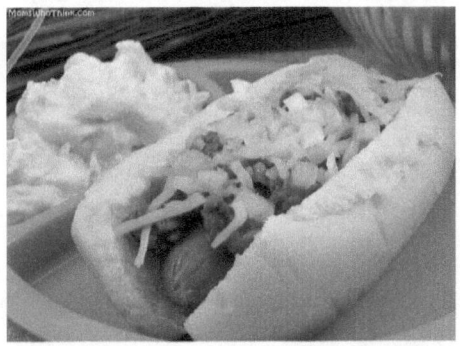

Looking for a show-stopping *dish* for lunch? Here's the chili dog's potato salad recipe to try out.

Ingredients

- 8 hot dog buns, split
- 8 hot dogs

- 1/4 teaspoon pepper
- 1 teaspoon salt
- 1 teaspoon hot pepper sauce
- 2 Tablespoons chili powder
- 1 can (6 ounces) tomato paste
- 1 cup tomato juice
- 1 garlic clove, minced
- 1-pound ground beef

Method

1. Cook garlic and beef in a large skillet over medium heat until the meat is no longer pink, drain. Stir in pepper, salt, pepper sauce, chili powder, tomato sauce, and tomato juice. Bring to boil.

2. Turn heat to medium low; simmer for 25 minutes. Serve while hot. Boil or grill hot dogs until heated through. Place it on buns and top with chili. Sprinkle with cheese and onion (if desired)

Tips/Notes

The chili dog potato salad is a great de-toxicant and antibiotic. Chili alone contains about 7 times more vitamin C than orange.

49. Pork Tenderloin Crispy Country Baked Beans

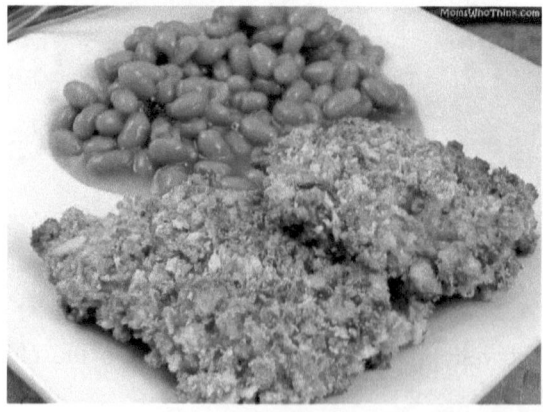

Pork tenderloin crispy cooked with mustard, butter and mayonnaise is a sweet dish and the results are very flavorful.

Ingredients

- 1 1/4 cups herb-seasoned (crushed) stuffing mix
- 4 to 5 teaspoons prepared mustard
- 1/4 cup mayonnaise
- 1/4 cup butter, melted
- 1-pound pork tenderloin cut cross-wise into 1-inch size medallions

Method

1. Flatten the pork tenderloin pieces to ¼ inch and ½ inch thickness. Combine mayonnaise, mustard and butter; add tenderloin pieces and roll in stuffing crumbs.

2. Place it in a greased 13 inches by 9 inches baking pan. Bake uncovered at 400 degrees F for about 15 minutes or until the juice is clear. Allow it to cool for 3 minutes before slicing.

Tips/Notes

Mayonnaise has several health benefits. It improves hair growth and contains vitamin E as well as oil content that keeps the heart healthy.

50. Country Baked Beans

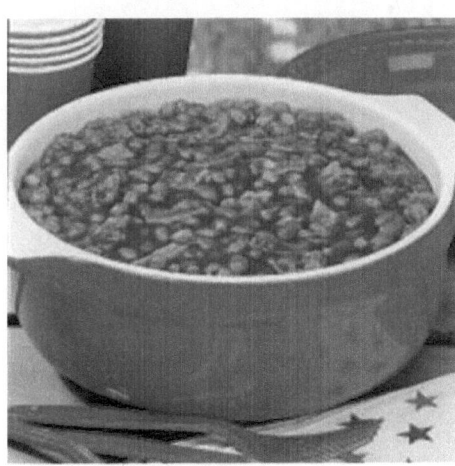

Nothing is more down-home than the flavorful country cooking, so it's only fitting that this recipe is one of the most delicious meals you can ever have for lunch.

Ingredients

- 1/2-pound bacon
- 1/2 cup catsup
- 1/2 cup brown sugar
- 1 teaspoon or more mustard
- 1 large can pork and beans

Method

1. Grease a large baking pan. Mix all the ingredients but bacon. Pour into the baking pan. Place the bacon strips on top. Cook for 40minutes at 350 degrees F.

Tips/Notes

Bacon and beans both have high levels of potassium and sodium. They also have a significant percentage of dietary fiber.

51. Cranberry Beef Buttered Corn Roast Baked Potatoes

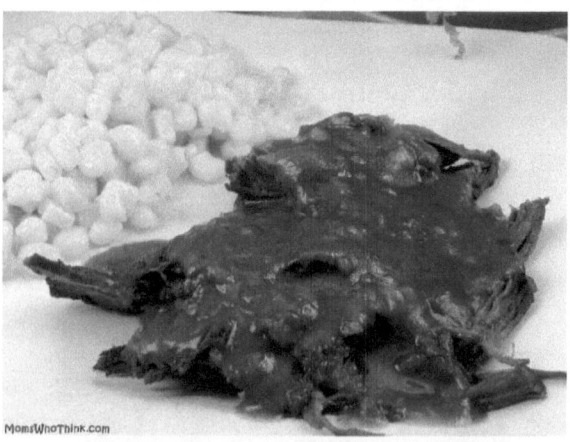

Beef chuck roast, onion soup mix and cranberry sauce will power your afternoon thanks to the nutritious and flavorful taste.

Ingredients

- 2 Tablespoons all-purpose flour
- 2 Tablespoons butter
- 1 (16 ounce) can jellied cranberry sauce

- 1 (3 pound) beef chuck roast
- 1 (1 ounce) envelope dry onion soup mix

Method

1. Place onion soup mix and roast in a slow cooker. Top it with cranberry sauce. Cover and cook on low heat. Remove roast, set it aside and set the slow cooker to high.

2. Whisk together flour and butter. Gently mix it with the liquid in the slow cooker to create thick gravy. Serve with buttered corn and baked potatoes.

Tips/Notes

The healthy benefits of cranberries include treatment of respiratory disorders, dental care, cancer as well as urinary tract conditions.

52. Baked Beans with Ham Cornbread

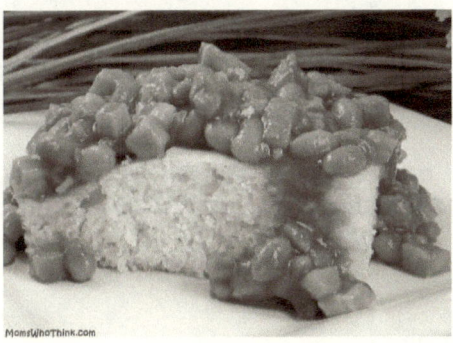

This recipe contains baked beans and ham and is sure to hit with its taco seasoning!

Ingredients

- 1 teaspoon minced fresh cilantro
- 1 teaspoon taco seasoning
- 1 teaspoon dried minced onion
- 1 Tablespoon Worcestershire sauce
- 1 Tablespoon brown sugar
- 2 Tablespoons molasses
- 1/4 cup tomato paste

- 2 cups cubed fully cooked ham
- 1 can (28 ounces) baked beans

Method

1. Combine all ingredients in a 1-½-qt. microwave bowl. Cover and microwave on high for 5 minutes until heated. Stir once and serve.

Tips/Notes

Ham contains vitamin B, particularly B1. It's also rich in proteins, magnesium and has the essential amino acids.

53. Cornbread

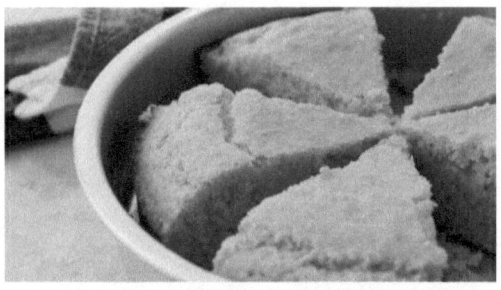

Take a good break from the regular bread with this mouthwatering fluffy cornbread. Cornbread for lunch? Yes, and you're going to love it!

Ingredients

- 1/2 cup vegetable oil
- 2 eggs
- 2/3 cup white sugar
- 1 teaspoon salt
- 1 Tablespoon baking powder
- 2 cups all-purpose flour
- 2 1/2 cups milk
- 1 1/2 cups cornmeal

Method

1. Pre-heat oven to 400 degrees F. Combine milk and corn meal. Let it stand for about 5 minutes.

2. Whisk together baking powder, flour, salt and sugar in a large bowl. Mix in oils, eggs and the cornmeal mixture until smooth. Pour butter into a prepared pan.

3. Bake in pre-heated oven for about 35 minutes or until a knife through the center of the cornbread comes out clean.

Tips/Notes

This recipe contains a little oil and tastes very good especially when served with the protein rich eggs and milk.

54. French Fries Cole Slaw Barbecued Beef Sandwiches

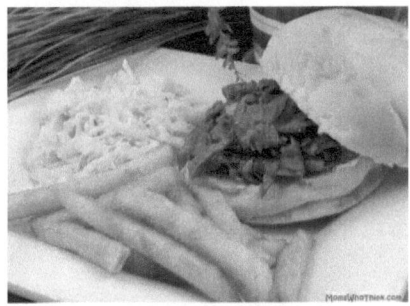

Enjoy with your choice of French fries, ground mustard, chopped onions and vinegar thanks to this fabulous recipe!

Ingredients

Barbecue Sauce

- 1 clove garlic, finely chopped
- 1/4 teaspoon ground mustard
- 2 teaspoons packed brown sugar
- 1 Tablespoon Worcestershire sauce
- 2 Tablespoons chopped onion
- 3 Tablespoons white vinegar
- 1/2 cup ketchup

Sandwiches

- 6 hamburger buns
- 1 lb. thinly-sliced cooked roast beef

- Cut it into 1-inch size strips (3 cups)
- Split

Method

1. Heat all sauce ingredients in a in a 1-quart saucepan. Bring to boil over medium heat. Stir constantly and reduce heat.

2. Simmer it uncovered for 10minutes, stirring occasionally. Stir the beef into sauce. Cover and simmer for about 4 minutes or until the beef is hot. Fill the buns with beef mixture. Serve with coleslaw and French fries (baked from frozen).

Tips/Notes

This recipe improves your cardiovascular health, preventing high cholesterol buildups.

55. KFC Coleslaw Recipe

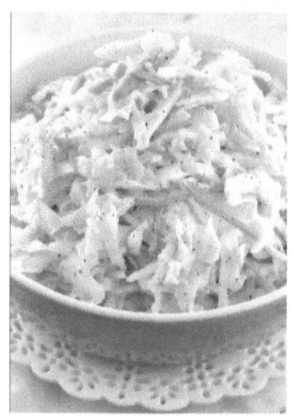

Virtually all KFC recipes are always flavorful and very delicious, and this one is just but the all-time favorite!

Ingredients

- 3 Tablespoons onions, dry minced
- 2 drops Tabasco
- 1/2 teaspoon celery seed
- 1/2 cup buttermilk
- 1/2 cup milk

- 1/4 teaspoon pepper
- 1/2 teaspoon salt
- 1 cup carrots, shredded
- 1/4 cup sugar
- 1 cabbage, shredded

Method

1. Slice the cabbage paper thin. Light toss with sugar and shredded carrots. Sprinkle with pepper and salt and drench it with milk. Cover and refrigerate for 10 minutes. Combine buttermilk, mayonnaise (not salad dressing), celery seed, minced onion and Tabasco.

2. Mix it well with the cabbage mixture. Refrigerate once more at least an hour before serving. Drain some of the dressing first before serving it separately at the table

Tips/Notes

Cabbage is ideal for weight loss! 1 cup of cooked cabbage contains about 33 calories. It's low in fat and amazingly high in fiber.

56. Perfect Mashed Potatoes

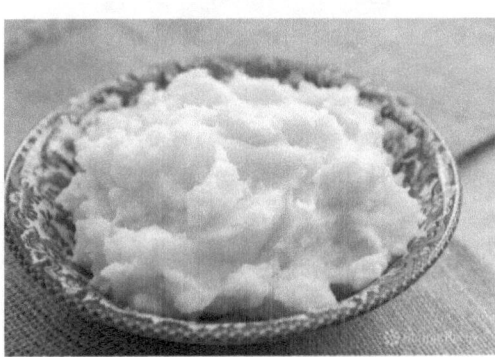

Heavenly mashed potatoes recipe using butter. You can't wait to prepare this dish!

Ingredients

- 2 Tablespoons chopped chives
- 3 Tablespoons butter
- 2 cups heavy cream

- Salt and pepper
- 4 pounds Yukon gold potatoes, peeled and cut into quarters

Method

1. Cook the potatoes. Add 2 Tablespoons salt and cover with cold water. Bring it to boil over medium heat. Cook until the potatoes become tender (about 20 minutes). Drain well. Put butter and cream in a small saucepan and heat.

2. Mash the potatoes well using a potato masher until smooth. Add the butter mixture/hot cream and season with pepper and salt. Mix well while adding the chives.

Tips/Notes

Mashed potatoes are a great benefit to the body. 1 cup of mashed potatoes contains about 622 milligrams of potassium.

57. Biscuit Pizza Casserole

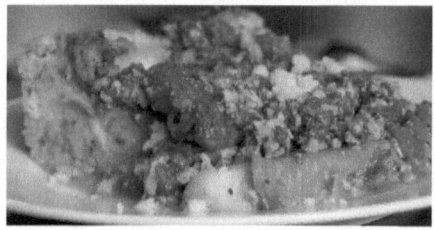

If you are a big fan of pizza and casserole then you're going to love this one!

Ingredients

- 2 cups shredded mozzarella cheese (8 oz.)
- 1 package (8 oz.) sliced pepperoni
- 2 cans (8 oz. each) pizza sauce (2 cups)
- 1 cup milk
- 3 1/3 cups Bisquick

Method

1. Pre-heat oven to 375 degrees F. Spray 3-quart glass baking dish with cooking spray.

2. In a bowl, stir the Bisquick mix and milk to form soft dough. Drop half of the dough using spoonful's over the bottom of the baking dish.

3. Sprinkle 1 can pizza sauce of dough. Scatter half of the pepperoni over sauce. Top with 1 cup of cheese. Repeat the rest of the layers with cheese, pepperoni, pizza sauce and dough. Bake until golden brown or for 25 minutes.

Tips/Notes

The biggest advantage of casseroles is that they are truly forgiving, allowing you the freedom to reduce or add ingredients as per your taste.

58. Blue Ribbon Chili Buttered Cornbread

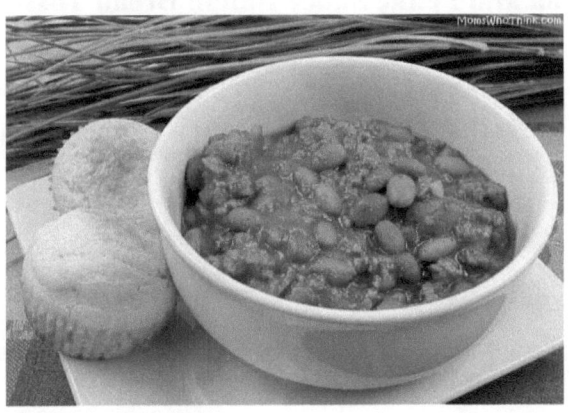

The recipe gets my vote for its quick and easy preparation without bargaining the flavors.

Ingredients

- 1 (15 ounce) can dark red kidney beans
- 1 (15 ounce) can light red kidney beans
- 4 Tablespoons chili seasoning mix
- 1 (8 ounce) jar salsa
- 2 1/2 cups tomato sauce
- 1/2 teaspoon garlic salt
- 1 teaspoon ground black pepper
- 1/2 onion, chopped
- 2 pounds ground beef

Method

1. Combine onion and ground beef in a saucepan and sauté for 15 minutes. Drain grease (if desired).

2. Add garlic salt, salsa, kidney beans, chili seasoning mix, tomato sauce and ground black pepper. Mix well, reducing heat to low. Simmer until meat and onion become tender. Serve

Tips/Notes

Black pepper has many health benefits such as relief from coughs, respiratory disorders, constipation, indigestion and impotency.

59. Vodka and Penne Sauce Italian Bread Tossed Salad

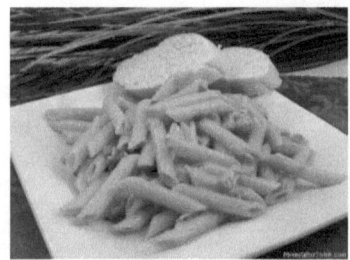

Sweet salty pancetta sautéed in butter and cooked in vodka, cream and tomato sauce makes a flavorful and rich sauce for boiled penne.

Ingredients

- 1/2 cup heavy whipping cream
- 1/4 pound chopped pancetta bacon
- 1/4 cup grated Parmesan cheese
- 1 1/2 cups tomato sauce
- 1/3 cup vodka
- 2 Tablespoons butter
- 1 (16 ounce) package penne pasta

Method

1. Bring water and salt to boil. Stir in pasta. Cook for 10 minutes and drain. Melt butter over medium heat. Add pancetta and sauté to light brown.

2. Add vodka and stir until it reduces to almost half (about 5 minutes). Stir in cream and tomato sauce. Simmer for 10 minutes. Stir frequently.

3. Add pasta and stir. Heat and serve with tossed salad, warm Italian bread and Parmesan cheese.

Tips/Notes

While vodka isn't exactly a health drink, it possesses valuable antiseptic, anti-bacterial qualities. It also reduces stress and boosts cardiovascular health.

60. Baked Corn

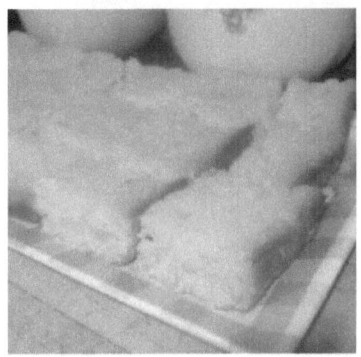

Here's a comforting recipe that should turn your ordinary lunches into something to celebrate!

Ingredients

- 1 (8.5 ounce) package dry corn muffin mix
- 2 eggs, beaten
- 3/4 cup melted butter
- 1 (8 ounce) container sour cream
- 1 (14.75 ounce) can cream-style corn
- 1 (15.25 ounce) can whole kernel corn, drained

Method

1. Pre-heat oven to 400 degrees F. Combine cream-style corn, whole-kernel corn, melted butter, eggs, sour cream and corn muffin mix. Mix well and pour it into one 9x13 inch baking pan. Bake for 30 minutes.

Tips/Notes

Corn protects the body from heart and cancer diseases thanks to its antioxidant activity.

61. Tater Tot Casserole Cornbread

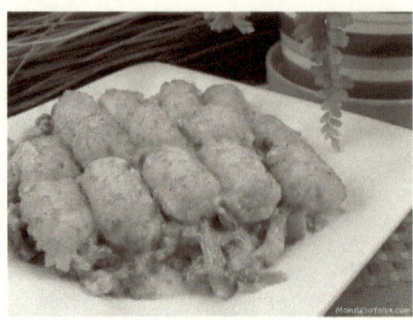

This is an easy and delicious dish loved by everyone and it's time to prepare it for lunch.

Ingredients

- 1 (32 ounce) package tater tots
- 1 (14.5 ounce) can French style green beans
- 1/2 teaspoon pepper
- 1 teaspoon salt
- 1 teaspoon garlic powder
- 1 cup whole milk
- 1 Can condensed cream of mushroom soup
- 1 (10.75 ounce) can condensed cream of chicken soup
- 1-pound ground beef

Method

1. Pre-heat oven to 350 degrees F. Brown the ground beef in a skillet, over high heat. Drain fat. Stir in green beans, pepper, salt, garlic powder, condensed cream of chicken soup, milk and condensed cream of mushroom soup.

2. Add the mixture into a medium sized casserole dish. Layer with tater tots. Bake in pre-heated oven for 30 minutes or until the tater tots become brown and crispy.

Tips/Notes

Packaged cornbread mix contains sugar.

62. Mozzarella Chicken Garlic Pasta Italian Bread

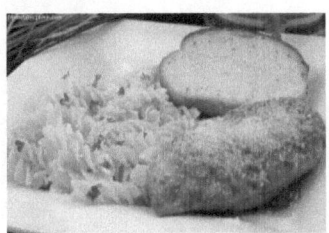

Mozzarella cheese, garlic, onion and chicken broth is a variation of Chicken Parmesan. This dish is served with hot cooked pasta, crusty Italian bread and salad.

Ingredients

- 1 cup shredded mozzarella cheese
- 4 cups spaghetti sauce
- 1/2 cup chicken broth
- 1/4 cup minced onion
- 1/2 teaspoon minced garlic
- 1/2 teaspoon ground black pepper
- 4 skinless, boneless chicken breast halves
- 1/2 Tablespoon olive oil

Method

1. Heat oil over medium heat. Sauté chicken breakfast for 4 minutes each side, until white. Add garlic, onion, pepper and broth.

2. Cover and simmer it over medium heat for 10 minutes (until broth cooks off). Stir in spaghetti. Cover and simmer for 10 more minutes. dSprinkle cheese over it and cover. Cook for another 3 minutes or until cheese is melted.

Tips/Notes

Thanks to this recipe's affordability and versatility it makes up a staple in the average diet.

63. Slow Cooker Pot Roast

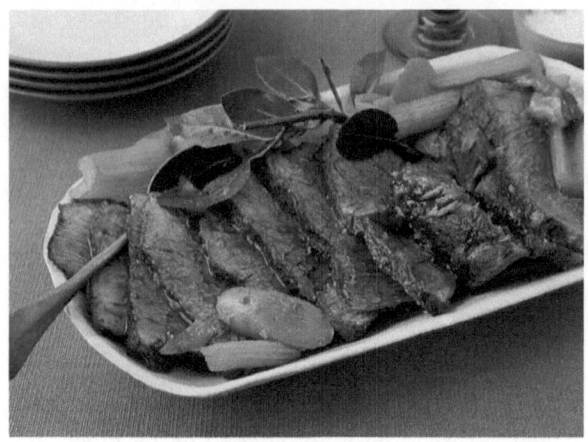

A paleo recipe for a crock pot roast with onions and mushrooms

Ingredients

- 2 cans condensed cream mushroom soup
- 5 1/2 pounds pot roast
- 1 1/4 cups water
- 1 (1 ounce) package dry onion soup mix

Method

1. Mix cream of mushroom soup, water and dry onion soup mix in a slow cooker. Put a pot roast in a slow cooker, coating it with soup mixture.

2. Cook on High heat. Serve it with buttered carrots and baked potatoes.

Tips/Notes

A pot roast is easy to prepare and makes a fabulous dish for lunch.

64. Saltine Fried Chicken Potato Salad Corn on the Cob

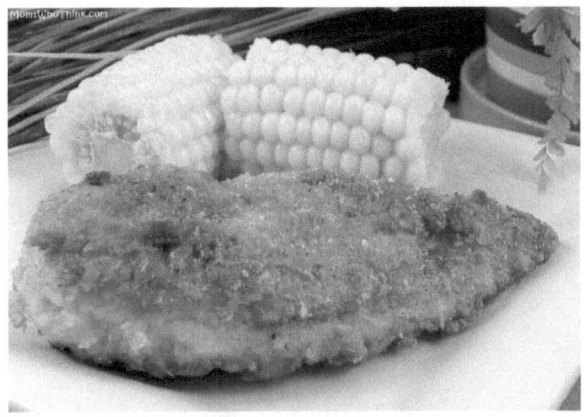

Here's another delicious recipe that combines chicken, corn and potatoes.

Ingredients

- 6 skinless, boneless chicken breast halves
- 1/4 cup vegetable oil
- 1 egg
- 1/2 teaspoon ground black pepper
- 1 teaspoon seasoned salt
- 2 Tablespoons dry potato flakes
- 2 Tablespoons all-purpose flour
- 30 saltine crackers

Method

1. Place crackers in a re-sealable plastic bag. Seal it and crush crackers to coarse crumbs. Add potato flakes, flour, pepper and seasoned salt to bag and mix. Beat egg in a dish.

2. Heat oil over medium-high heat and dredge chicken pieces one after another in egg beat. Place it in bag with the crumb mixture. Seal the bag and shake to coat. Reduce the heat to medium and cook coated chicken in skillet for 15-20 minutes, frequently turning it until golden brown

Tips/Notes

This dish tastes as good as it looks!

65. Brown Sugar Kielbasa Twice Baked Potatoes

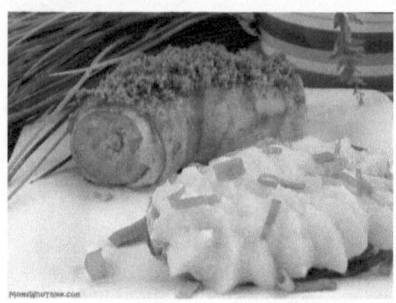

Twice baked potatoes are too hearty to stand alone and therefore combine brown sugar, kielbasa and bacon.

Ingredients

- 1 cup brown sugar
- 1-pound bacon
- 1 (16 ounce) package kielbasa

Method

1. Pre-heat oven to 375 degrees F. Slice the bacon into halves, wrapping each strip around the kielbasa. Place on a baking sheet and sprinkle liberally with brown sugar. Bake until the bacon becomes crisp and the brown sugar is melted.

Tips/Notes

Kielbasa offers a high level of protein per serving.

66. Onion Roasted Potatoes Salisbury steak Corn on the Cob

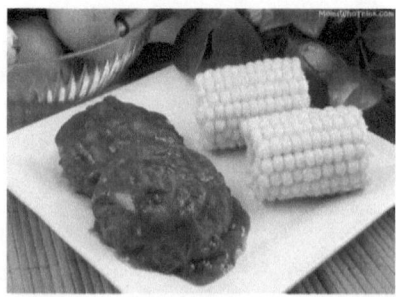

This recipe contains bread crumbs, ground beef, egg and meat. Mustard powder and black paper takes the flavor to another level.

Ingredients

- 1/2 teaspoon mustard powder
- 1 Tablespoon Worcestershire sauce
- 1/4 cup water
- 1/4 cup ketchup
- 1 Tablespoon all-purpose flour
- 1/8 teaspoon ground black pepper
- 1/4 teaspoon salt
- 1 egg
- 1/2 cup dry bread crumbs
- 1 1/2 pounds ground beef
- 1 can condensed onion soup

Method

1. Mix together ground beef, bread crumbs, ⅓ cup condensed French onion soup, black pepper, egg, and salt. Shape into 6 oval patties. Over medium heat, brown both sides of patties in a skillet. Drain fat.

2. Blend the remaining soup and flour in a bowl until smooth. Mix in water, ketchup, mustard powder and Worcestershire sauce. Pour it over meat in the skillet. Cover and cook for 15 minutes, stirring occasionally and serve.

Tips/Notes

Mustard powder offers amazing cancer fighting benefits.

67. Rosemary Lemon Chicken

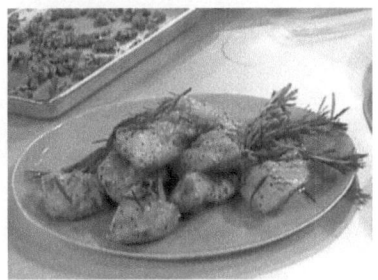

This recipe uses an easy made marinade with lemon juice and rosemary that makes it a delightfully flavorful dish!

Ingredients

- 1 teaspoon black pepper
- 1 teaspoon salt
- 1 lemon, sliced
- 1 tablespoon rosemary, dried
- 3 tablespoons olive oil
- 4 large chicken thighs, bone-in, skin-on

Method

1. Place chicken thighs in a dish. Drizzle over the lemon slices, rosemary, olive oil, salt and pepper. Cover and let it marinate in the refrigerator for 25 minutes.

2. Preheat the oven to 400 degrees F. Preheat a cast iron pan over medium-high heat.

3. When hot, drain the chicken breasts of excess oil. Place in chicken thigh in the pan, skin side down. Bake for 20 minutes and let it cool before serving.

Tips/Notes

Rosemary has a memorable flavor and offers unique health benefits that make it an indispensable herb for every kitchen. It also has anti-oxidant qualities.

68. Speedy Mediterranean chicken

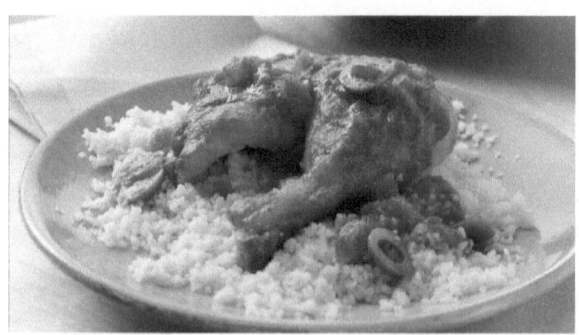

This dinner recipe combines sweet raisins, honey, chunky salsa and curry powder for a little bit of sugar and spice!

Ingredients

- 1/4 cup honey
- 1 deli rotisserie chicken (2 to 2 1/2 lb.), cut into 6 to 8 pieces, skin removed if desired
- 1/4 cup golden raisins
- 1/2 cup sliced green olives
- 1 jar salsa
- 2 teaspoons curry powder
- 1 tablespoon olive or vegetable oil

Method

1. Heat oil over medium heat in a 12-inch non-stick skillet. Stir in curry powder and cook over medium heat for 60 seconds. Stir constantly, adding the remaining ingredients but chicken.

2. Add chicken and turn to coat. Turn heat to medium high. Cover and cook for 5 minutes and serve.

Tips/Notes

Raisins are great sources of antioxidants, dietary fiber, and vitamins. Salsa is also a great anti-oxidant.

69. Seafood Bake

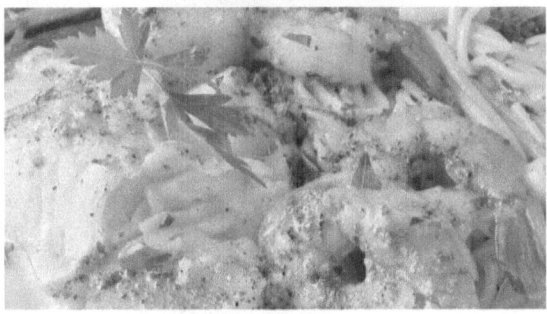

Talk of halibut fillets, scallops and shrimp combined—my mouth is watering already!

Ingredients

- 1 tablespoon chopped fresh parsley
- Salt and pepper to taste
- 1 teaspoon minced garlic
- 1/2 teaspoon seafood seasoning
- 1 tablespoon lemon juice
- 2 tablespoons melted butter
- 1/3 cup dry white wine
- 6 peeled and deveined jumbo shrimps, tail still attached
- 6 scallops
- 2 (4 ounce) halibut fillets

Method

1. Pre-heat oven to 400 degrees F. Arrange the shrimp, scallops and halibut in an oven safe baking dish. Drizzle with lemon juice, butter and wine. Sprinkle garlic.

2. Season to taste with pepper and salt. Bake in pre-heated oven for 10-12 minutes. Sprinkle with parsley and serve.

Tips/Notes

Shrimps are rich in heart healthy Omega-3's than most types of fish.

70. Easy Chicken Lo Mein

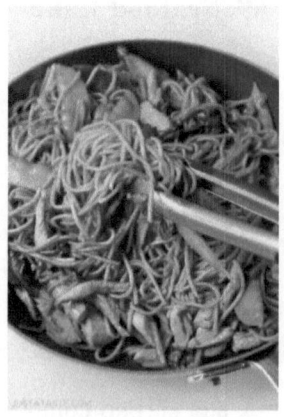

This recipe is not only budget-friendly but it's also very yummy. Talk of an easy and cheap fabulous dinner!

Ingredients

- 1/4 cup water
- 1 1-lb bag frozen mixed oriental vegetables
- 1 3-ounce package chicken flavor ramen noodle soup
- 2 teaspoons freshly grated ginger or 1 teaspoon powder
- 2 tablespoons soy sauce or teriyaki sauce
- 1 clove garlic, minced
- 1 lb. boneless skinless chicken breast, cut into thin slices
- 1 tablespoon oil-sesame or peanut oil

Method

1. Heat oil over medium heat until hot. Add chicken and stir. Add vegetables and cover. Cook for 5 minutes.

2. Meanwhile, cook the noodles according to package directions. Drain. Add soy sauce, ginger, garlic and seasoning packet to water. Mix and over vegetables and chicken. Add the noodles and toss to mix. Serve

Tips/Notes

Both peanut and sesame oil are very helpful in achieving radiant health, a flawless skin and healthier hair from the inside out.

71. Apples Candied Sweet Potatoes with Pork Chops Dinner Rolls

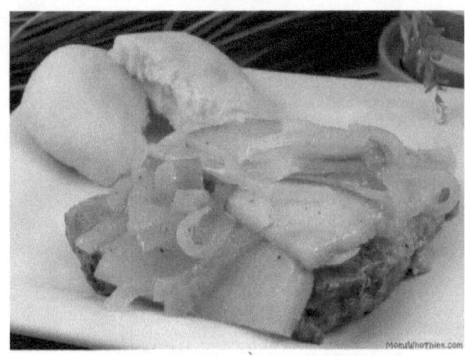

This is yet another very delicious yet easy to prepare dinner meal. Apples, sweet potatoes and pork chops. What a hearty meal for dinner!

Ingredients

- 4 bone-in pork loin chops
- 1 Tablespoon brown sugar
- 2 Tablespoons honey mustard
- 1 large red apple, cut into thin wedges
- 1 large green apple, cut into thin wedges
- 2 medium onions, thinly sliced
- 1/4 teaspoon pepper
- 1/4 teaspoon salt
- 2 Tablespoons vegetable oil

Method

1. Using oil on each side, brown pork chops in a large skillet and season with pepper and salt. Remove and keep warm. In the same skillet, sauté apple wedges and onions until crisp-tender. Combine brown sugar and mustard. Brush over chops. Return to the skillet and cook for 5 minutes or until meat juices clear.

Tips/Notes

Sweet potatoes are extremely versatile and very healthy. They help fight cancer, get stronger bones and control your diabetes.

72. Barbecued Baby Back Ribs

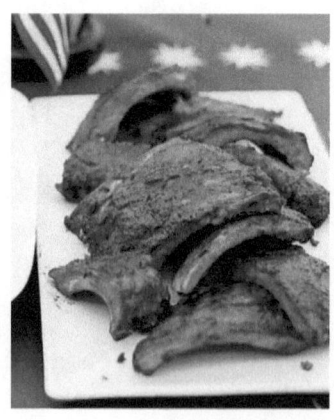

If you are a meat lover then this easy dinner is definitely going to please you!

Ingredients

- 1 cup barbecue sauce, divided
- 2 (about 4 pounds total) racks pork baby back ribs

Method

1. Pre-heat oven to 400 degrees F. Place the rack of ribs on a piece of aluminum foil (should be large enough to completely wrap the ribs).

2. Brush the ribs with ½ barbecue sauce and wrap tightly in foil. Place this on rimmed baking sheets. Bake until fork-tender.

3. Unwrap the ribs and return them to baking sheets and brush the remaining barbecue sauce. Cover. Preheat boiler and cook until sauce begins to brown. Cut them into individual ribs and serve

Tips/Notes

Meat is the leading source of proteins and amino acids so you want to have a really cool grab during breakfast.

73. Chili-rubbed Tilapia with Lemon and Asparagus

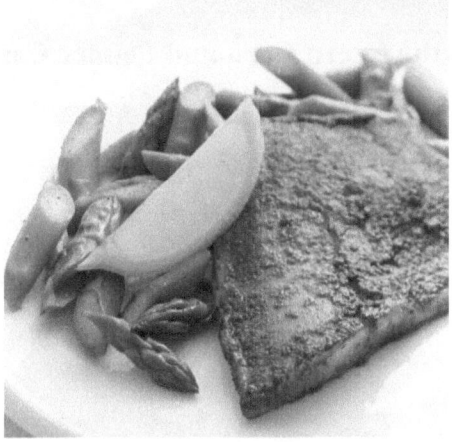

This recipe features protein packed fish—a favorite of many. It's sure to hit with its citrus, chili and garlic flavors.

Ingredients

- 3 tablespoons lemon juice
- 2 tablespoons extra-virgin olive oil
- 1-pound tilapia
- 1/2 teaspoon salt, divided
- 1/2 teaspoon garlic, powder
- 2 tablespoons chili powder
- 2 (trimmed) pounds asparagus

Method

1. Bring 1 inch of water to boil in a saucepan. Place asparagus in a steamer basket, put in the saucepan. Steam for about 5 minutes. Transfer to a plate and let it cool. Combine garlic powder, ¼ teaspoon salt and chili powder. Dredge the fillets spice mixture and heat over medium high.

2. Add fish and cook for about 5 minutes. Add lemon juice, salt and asparagus to the pan and cook. Stir constantly until the asparagus is heated through and coated (2 minutes). Serve the asparagus with fish.

Tips/Notes

Give an almighty punch to heart related diseases and cancer with the help of asparagus contained in this recipe.

74. Southwestern Corn and Pepper Casserole

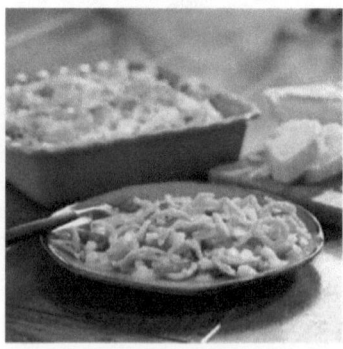

This delectable dinner recipe contains casseroles, milk, corn, cheese, zesty peppers in a mouthwatering cheese sauce!

Ingredients

- 2/3 cups French's Cheddar French Fried Onions
- 2/3 cup shredded Mexican blend cheese
- 1/3 teaspoon Pepper Sauce (optional)
- 1/2 cup milk
- 1, 10 3/4-ounce Can Campbell's Southwestern Pepper Jack Soup or Cheddar Cheese Soup
- 1, 10-ounce package frozen whole kernel corn
- 2 cups frozen peppers and onions for stir-fry

Method

1. Combine onions, corn and pepper in a 1 ½ quart microwave safe casserole. Cover. Microwave on high heat for 8 minutes, stirring through cooking.

2. Drain and stir in milk, soup, 2/3 cup French Fried Onions, 1/3 cup cheese and Frank's Red-hot Sauce. Sprinkle with the remaining onions and cheese. Bake at 350 degrees F for 20 minutes. Serve.

Tips/Notes

Corn contains two elements zeaxanthin and lutein that promote a healthy vision.

75. Fennel Crusted Sirloin

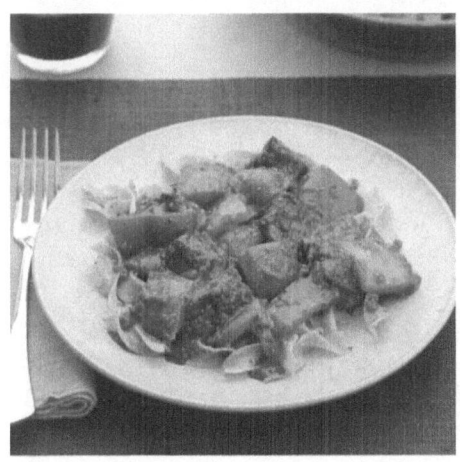

Who can resist sirloin? This fabulous dish is a pure comfort, featuring tender meat and gravy. This is an ideal meal to fuel you through the afternoon.

Ingredients

- 1 tablespoon all-purpose flour
- Freshly ground pepper
- 2 bell peppers
- 1/4 cup dry red wine
- 3/4 cup divided non-sodium beef broth
- 1 tablespoon minced garlic
- 1 tablespoon extra-virgin olive oil
- 1/2 teaspoon kosher salt, divided
- 1 teaspoon fennel seed, coarsely ground or roughly chopped
- 8-ounce sirloin steak trimmed of fat and sliced into 1-inch chunks

Method

1. Rub steak with ¼ teaspoon salt. Heat oil over medium high heat. Add the steak and cook until browned. Transfer it to a plate and cover it with foil to keep warm. Add garlic and cook (about 30 seconds).

2. Add broth, wine bell peppers, teaspoon salt and pepper; bring to simmer, cover and reduce heat. Cook for 5 more minutes. Whisk the remaining flour and 1/4 cup broth in a bowl. Add it to the pepper mixture.

3. Return the steak to the pan. Turn heat to low simmer. Cook for another 2 minutes for medium rare.

Tips/Notes

Sirloin steak is a rich source of protein.

76. Easy Chicken Taco Salad

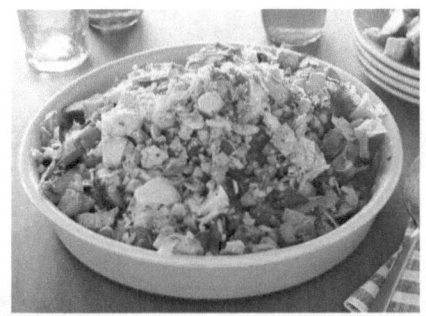

If its midweek and you aren't too hungry but still want a tasty meal to munch on, why not try the taco salad?

Ingredients

- 1 package tortilla chips
- Cheddar cheese, shredded (fresh or packaged)
- 1 bag mixed salad green
- 1/2 package taco seasoning
- 1/2 can salsa
- 1 whole chicken breast

Method

1. Sauté chicken in a fry pan (use a little oil so chicken doesn't stick). Once cooked, remove from pan and dice up the chicken. Add Taco seasoning and salsa.

2. Place chicken diced to pan and simmer in sauce for 25 minutes. Place lettuce on a plate and add Taco mix on top of lettuce. Serve with chips on the side

Tips/Notes

Tacos recipes help keep the calorie count to the minimum.

77. Honey Pecan Pork Cutlets

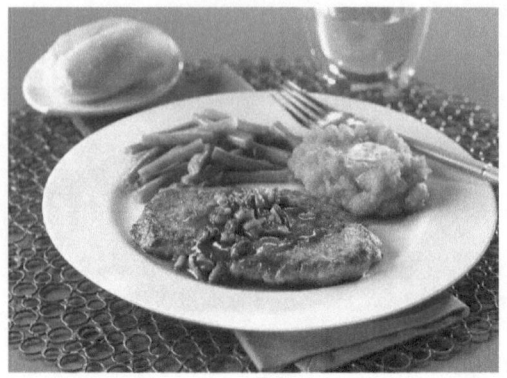

Are you aware that pork has an equal amount of proteins (22 grams) as most fish filets? If you haven't tried pork before, here's your chance.

Ingredient

- 1/4 cup chopped pecans
- 1/4 cup honey
- 3 tablespoons butter
- Flour for dredging
- 1-pound pork loin cutlets pounded to 1/4-inch thickness

Method

1. Dredge the cutlets in flour. Heat butter over medium heat. Add cutlets and sauté for 5 minutes. Mix the remaining butter with pecans and honey. Add to skillet and stir. Cover and simmer for 7 minutes. Spoon any remaining pecans and sauce over the cutlets and serve.

Tips/Notes

Pork is a great source of protein.

78. Garlicky Steak

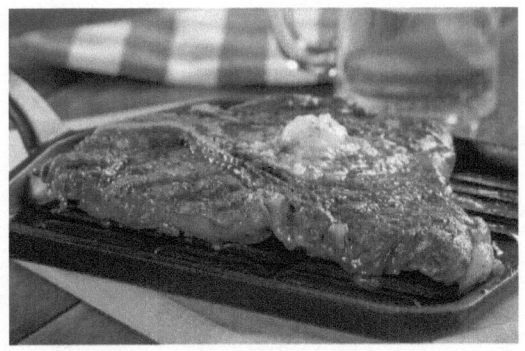

This recipe contains fresh garlic to really spruce up the flavor of a T-bone steak!

Ingredients

- 1 tablespoon fresh parsley
- 1 tablespoon chopped garlic
- 1/4 cup (1/2 stick) butter
- 1/4 teaspoon black pepper
- 1/4 teaspoon salt
- 2 (12-ounce) T-bone steaks

Method

1. Season steaks with pepper and salt. Using a grill pan, brown steaks over medium high heat for 3 minutes. Remove the pan from heat. Turn heat to low. Add garlic, parsley, and butter. Cook for 2 minutes and serve immediately.

Tips/Notes

Garlic has great anti-viral, anti-bacterial, anti-oxidant and anti-fungal properties.

79. Curried Chicken Salad

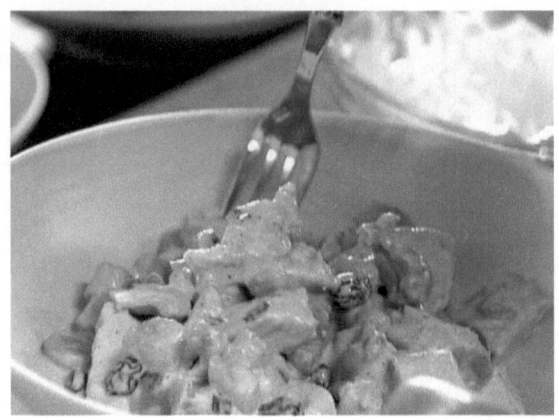

Curried chicken salad recipe is a lightly spiced, fruit salad that's a better take on Coronation chicken.

Ingredients

- 1 tbsp. cilantro (chopped)
- 1/4 cup grapes (halved)
- 1/8 cup red onion (diced)
- 1/2 cup roasted chicken (diced)
- 1/4 tbsp. curry powder
- Mixed greens
- 2 tbsp. nonfat plain Greek yogurt

Method

1. Combine nonfat plain Greek yogurt and curry powder. Add roasted chicken, diced red onion, grapes and chopped cilantro. Top with a handful mixed greens.

Tips/Notes

Chicken supplies a good amount of protein, essential vitamins and minerals. It also helps tame cholesterol levels.

80. Mango Quesadillas

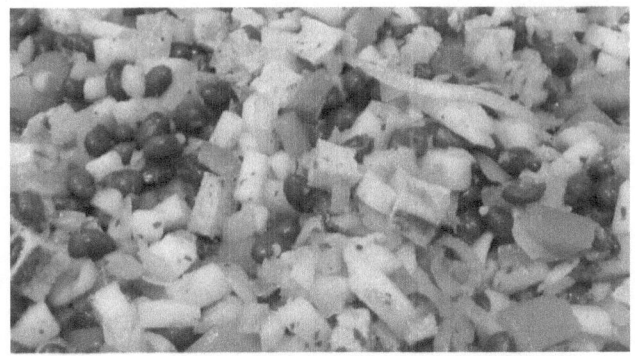

This recipe proves that sweet spicy and savory work together perfectly!

Ingredients

- 1 tbsp. scallion (chopped)
- 1/8 cup crumbled queso fresco or feta cheese
- 2 slices deli ham
- 1/8 cup mango chutney
- 1 8-inch, whole-wheat tortilla

Method

1. Spread mango chutney with whole wheat tortilla. Add scallion (chopped), 2 slices deli ham, crumbled queso fresco or feta cheese.

2. Fold in half and grill for 4 minutes on each side. Cut into quarters and enjoy.

Tips/Notes

Mangoes are perfect for fighting cancer and regulating diabetes. They alkaline the body, help in digestion and clean the skin.

81. Fancy Fig Sandwich

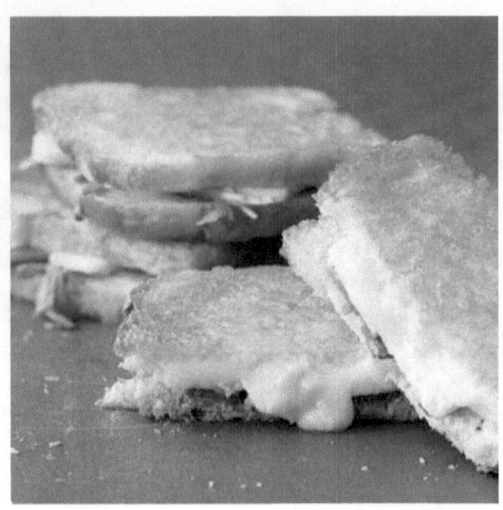

This is a very tasty and easy to prepare dinner recipe.

Ingredients

- 1 tsp. thinly sliced basil
- 2 tsp. fig preserves
- Whole-grain bread
- Lemon zest
- 1/2 tsp. honey
- 2 slices goat cheese

Method

1. Mix together honey, goat cheese and a pinch lemon zest. Spread the mixture between slices of whole grain bread. Add thinly sliced basil and preserves.

2. Grill the sandwich in a pan for 4 minutes or prepare in a Panini press until warmed through.

Tips/Notes

Even without toppings, sandwich delivers a good amount of proteins, 10 times more than your daily intake of 11 minerals and vitamins.

82. Low-Carb Roll-Up

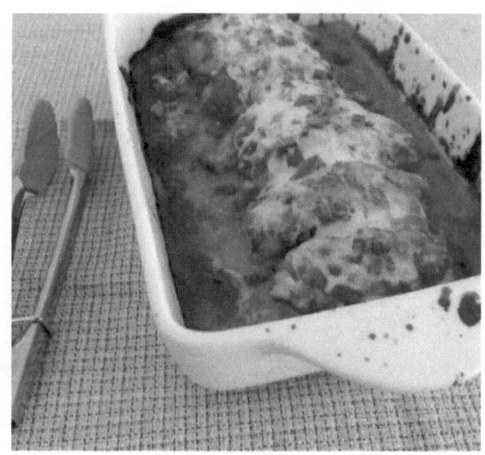

My best low Carb snack or diner option is the "no bread" roll ups.

Ingredients

- 2 slices avocado
- 1 tablespoon pesto (store-bought or homemade)
- 1 slice provolone cheese
- 1 slice low-sodium deli turkey

Method

1. Layer provolone cheese and low-sodium deli turkey on a plate. Spread the cheese with pesto (store bought or homemade!).

2. Top with 2 slices avocado. Roll up the turkey and repeat two more times.

Tips/Notes

Also known as butter fruit/alligator pear, avocado is the only fruit that delivers a significant amount of healthy fats (monounsaturated fat).

83. Black Bean Wrap

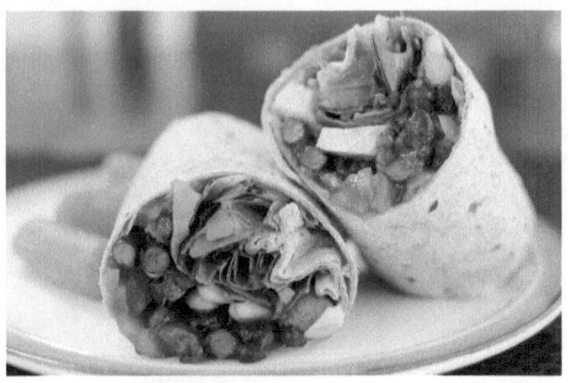

Black beans whole wheat bread is super healthy and unbelievably full of.

Ingredients

- 2 tablespoon salsa
- 1 tbsp. cheddar cheese
- A pinch of paprika
- A pinch of cumin
- 1/4 cup black beans (drained and rinsed)
- 1/8-inch whole-wheat bread

Method

1. Mash drained and rinsed black beans on whole-wheat bread using a fork.

2. Sprinkle with a pinch of paprika, cumin and cheddar cheese. Roll up and microwave for 40 seconds. Serve with salsa.

Tips/Notes

Cumin present in this recipe aids in digestion, treats piles, respiratory disorders, bronchitis, and asthma therefore improving the immune system.

84. Loaded Sweet Potato

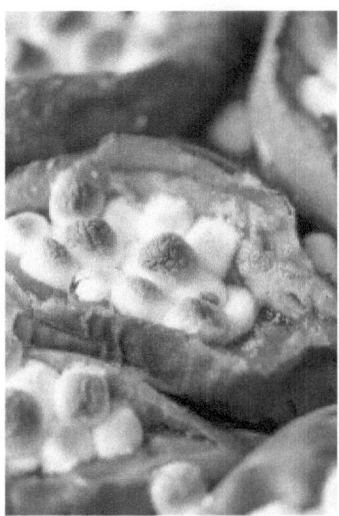

Loaded sweet potato should indeed be LOADED. It contains black beans, onions, potato and honey.

Ingredients

- 2 tablespoons drained and rinsed black beans
- 1 tsp. honey
- 2 tablespoon nonfat Greek yogurt
- A pinch of paprika
- 1 sweet potato

Method

1. Prick the sweet potato with a fork (4-5 times). Microwave it on a microwave-safe plate or paper towel for 5 minutes.

2. Split open and top with nonfat Greek yogurt, a pinch of paprika, drained and rinsed beans and honey. Serve.

Tips/Notes

Sweet potatoes nutrients help prevent oxidative damage to our cells.

85. Green Tortilla Pizza

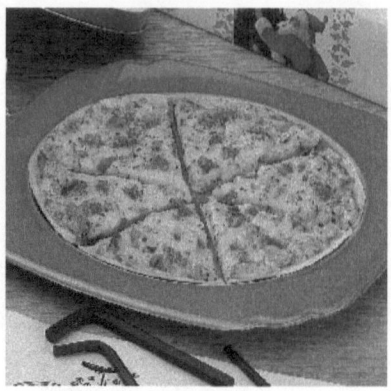

A super easy individual pizza made with mushrooms, tortilla, tomato sauce and spinach.

Ingredients

- 2 tablespoons part-skim mozzarella
- 2 tablespoons chopped onions
- 4 sliced baby bella mushrooms
- A large handful of spinach
- 2 tablespoons chopped broccoli florets
- 1 whole-grain 8-inch tortilla
- 2 tablespoons pesto (homemade or store bought)

Method

1. Pre-heat boiler to 350 degrees F. Spread pesto on whole grain tortilla.

2. Sprinkle with the 4-sliced baby bella mushrooms, a large handful of spinach, part-skim mozzarella, chopped onions and chopped broccoli florets.

3. Broil until cheese is browned (about 5 minutes).

Tips/Notes

Tortilla is very nutritious and is rich in phosphorous content; a very critical component of health tissue.

86. Souper Spicy Soup

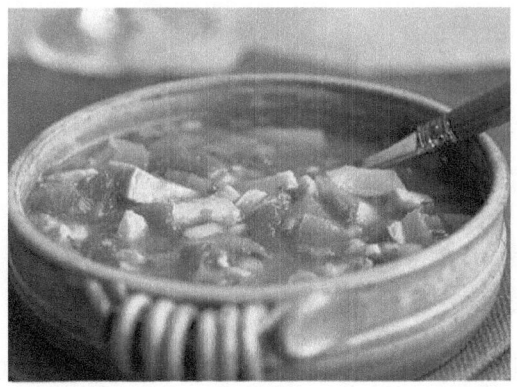

Every culture has its own favorite spicy soup but this one stands tall.

Ingredients

- 1/4 cup broccoli
- 1/4 cup chopped cauliflower
- 1/8 cup uncooked couscous
- 1/2 tbsp. olive oil
- Crushed red pepper flakes
- 3/4 cup vegetable broth
- 1 (thinly sliced) scallion
- 1 oil-packed sun-dried tomato (chopped)

Method

1. Combine vegetable broth, olive oil and a pinch of crushed red pepper flakes.

2. When it comes to boil, stir in chopped cauliflower, broccoli and uncooked couscous.

3. Cook until tender and top with thinly sliced scallion and oil-packed sun-dried tomato.

Tips/Notes

Cauliflower nutrients prevent mutations and help reduce stress from free radicals.

87. Hawaiian Wrap

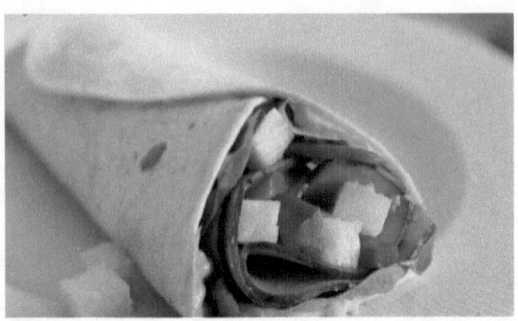

This recipe totally satisfied the urge I had for pineapple, carrots, cage, ham, yogurt all combined.

Ingredients

- 1/8-inch, whole-wheat tortilla
- 1/4 cup nonfat Greek yogurt
- 1/4 head Napa cabbage
- 2 slices of deli ham (chopped)
- A handful of vegetables
- 1/2 carrots (shredded)
- 1/4 cup pineapple (diced)
- 1/2 tsp. caraway seeds
- 1 tbsp. white wine vinegar

Method

1. Combine tablespoon caraway seeds, white wine vinegar and nonfat Greek yogurt in a bowl.

2. Toss together thinly sliced Napa cabbage, deli ham, shredded carrot, and pineapple.

3. Dress vegetables with Greek yogurt mixture and roll it in a whole wheat wrap tortilla.

Tips/Notes

Pineapple is a winner when it comes to boosting your immune system, cleansing the body and nourishing hair.

88. Grilled Cheddar n' Apple

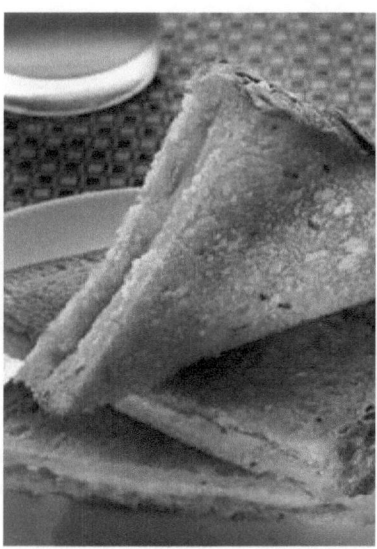

It's dinner time! You know what that means: It's time for a really hearty meal!

Ingredients

- 1 tablespoon deli mustard
- 1/2 green apple (thinly sliced)
- 1 to 2 slices sharp cheddar cheese
- 2 slices of whole-grain bread

Method

1. Layer 1/2 thinly sliced green apple and slices of sharp cheddar cheese between slices of whole grain bread.

2. Spread one slice of bread with 1 tablespoon deli mustard. Grill in a nonstick pan for 3 minutes on each side. Cook in a Panini press until cheese is completely melted.

Tips/Notes

For matters related to bone strength and health issues such as osteoporosis, cheddar is a winner!

89. Lighter Chef's Salad

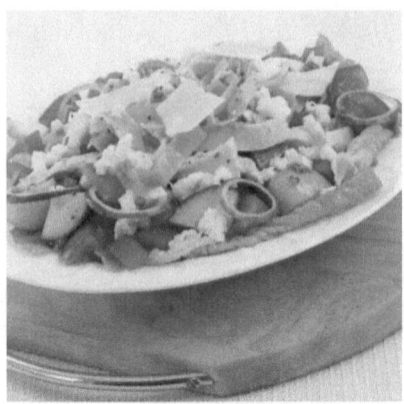

Lighter Chef's salad with turkey, romaine lettuce and avocado is a really tasty dish! Toss together this mouthwatering salad for a dinner dish that won't let you down!

Ingredients

- 1/8 shaved Parmesan
- 1/4 head of romaine lettuce (cut into bite size pieces)
- 1/4 sliced red onion
- 2 slices deli turkey
- 1/2 avocado (cut into bite-sized pieces)
- 1/2 sliced tomato
- 1 tablespoon balsamic vinegar
- Salt

Method

1. Tear head of romaine lettuce into bite-sized pieces.

2. Top lettuce with shaved Parmesan, sliced red onion, slices deli turkey, avocado (cut into bite-sized pieces), sliced tomato, balsamic vinegar, salt and pepper to taste. Serve.

Tips/Notes

Romaine lettuce is rich in anti-oxidants, minerals and vitamins such as A, manganese and folate.

90. Open-Faced White Bean Sandwich

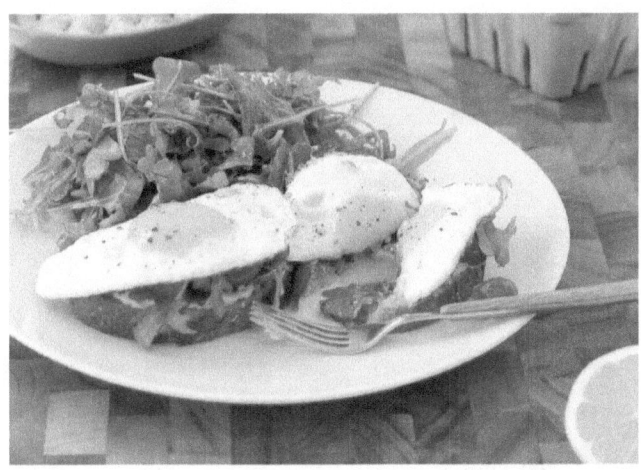

A healthy dinner time meal prepared with white beans, cucumber slices, olive oil and whole grain bread.

Ingredients

- 1/4 can rinsed and drained white beans
- Whole-grain bread
- 1 tablespoon olive oil
- 1 slice red onion
- A pinch of salt and pepper
- 1/4 avocado (sliced)
- 5 cucumber slices

Method

1. Mash rinsed and drained white beans with olive oil and a pinch of pepper and salt.

2. Toast a slice of whole grain bread, spreading with the bean mixture. Top with cucumber slices, avocado and red onion.

Tips/Notes

Cucumber aids in hydration, decreases irritation and swelling of the skin thanks to the presence of vitamin K.

91. Roast Beef Roll

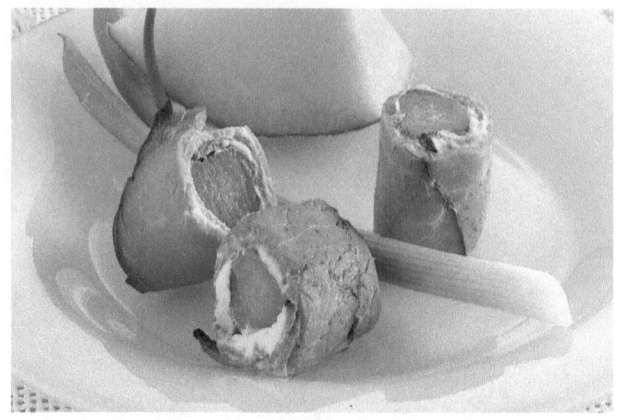

Serve up a spectacular centerpiece of roast beef with cheddar, romaine lettuce and whole wheat wrap.

Ingredients

- A handful of romaine lettuce
- 1 Oz sliced cheddar
- 2 Oz Roast beef
- 1 whole wheat wrap
- 1/2 tablespoon horseradish
- 1 Oz light cream cheese

Method

1. Spread horseradish and Oz cream cheese on whole wheat wrap.

2. Layer a handful of romaine lettuce, sliced cheddar, and roast beef. Roll up and enjoy!

Tips/Notes

The presence of horseradish in this recipe offers treatment for hypertension, chest related problems and chronic heart failure.

92. Niçoise Sandwich

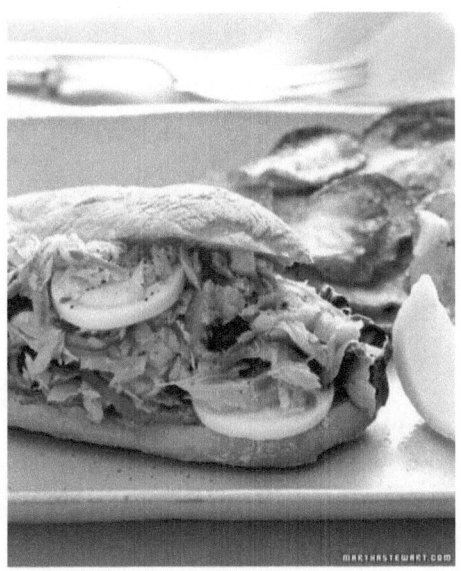

The Niçoise recipe comes with tuna, spinach, black olives and whole wheat baguette, all combined so you don't get bored.

Ingredients

- 1/4 whole-wheat baguette (4 inches in length)
- 1 tbsp. olive oil
- 1/4 cup pitted black olives (chopped)
- 1/4 cup halved cherry tomatoes
- Baby spinach leaves
- 1/6-oz Can tuna

Method

1. Combine halved cherry tomatoes, pitted black olives, tuna and olive oil.

2. Split open whole wheat baguette and fill with baby spinach leaves and the tuna mixture. Serve.

Tips/Notes

Black olives have anti-oxidant qualities that impede oxidation of cholesterol.

93. Mediterranean Pita

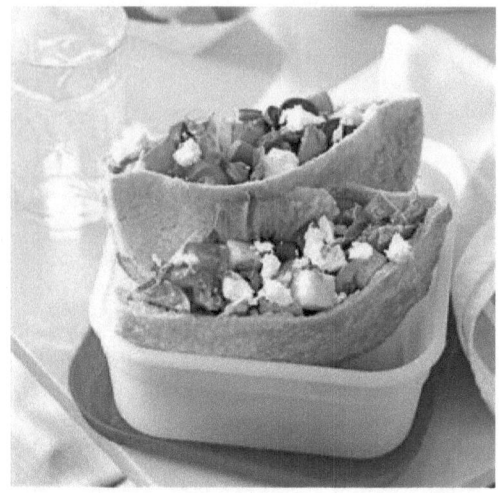

A one of a kind dinner time! Expect a fabulous meal, and the personal touch this meal has to offer.

Ingredients

- 1 large roasted red pepper
- A handful of mixed greens
- Whole wheat pita
- 2 tablespoons hummus
- 1 tablespoon crumbled feta
- 5 cucumber slices
- 1 tablespoon black olives

Method

1. Split open whole wheat pita. Spread with hummus.

2. Add crumbled feta, roasted red pepper (preferably sliced) cucumber, black olives and a handful of mixed greens. Serve.

Tips/Notes

Hummus is the unique ingredient in this recipe. It improves the digestive system, muscular and cardiovascular health functions.

94. Taco Salad

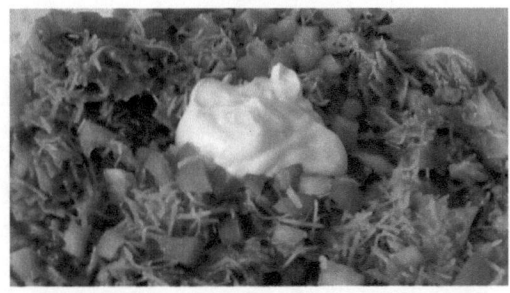

Not only is the taco salad easy to prepare, it's also super filling!

Ingredients

- 1 chopped scallion
- 2 tablespoons salsa
- 1 tablespoon chili powder
- 1 tablespoon olive oil
- 1 tablespoon low fat Greek yogurt
- 1/2 thinly sliced celery stalk
- 1/4 cup drained and rinsed black beans
- 2 tablespoons corn
- 1 tablespoon chopped black olives
- 2 cups baby spinach
- Lightly toasted tortilla (optional)

Method

1. Combine low fat Greek yogurt, salsa, chili powder and olive oil for the dressing.

2. Serve dressing over a salad with drained and rinsed black beans, corn, chopped black olives, chopped scallion, thinly sliced celery stalk and baby spinach.

3. Add lightly toasted tortilla sliced into strips to each salad (optional). Serve.

Tips/Notes

Greek yogurt helps lose weight and fend off a cold.

95. Quinoa Salad

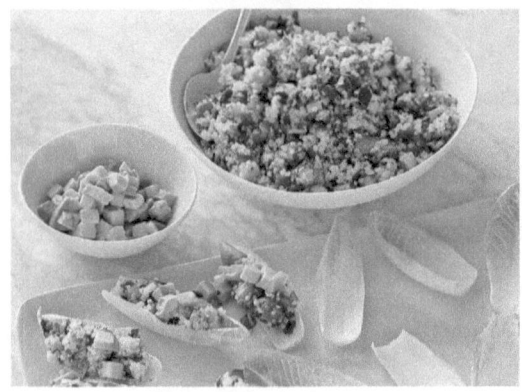

This is a flavorful, healthy salad that combines quinoa with lemon juice, chick peas and tuna.

Ingredients

- 1 tsp. lemon juice
- 1 tbsp. olive oil
- 1 tbsp. chopped parsley
- 1/4 cup rinsed and drained chick peas
- 1/2 Can tuna (optional)
- 1/2 cup rinsed quinoa
- 1 cup water
- 2 tablespoons chopped bell pepper

Method

1. Microwave rinsed quinoa and water at high heat for 5 minutes. Reduce to medium high and microwave for another 5 minutes.

2. Fluff and stir in rinsed and drained chick peas, chopped parsley, chopped bell pepper, lemon juice, olive oil, pepper and salt to taste.

3. Add tuna for a meatier dinner meal (optional). Serve.

Tips/Notes

Want to be lavished with anti-inflammatory and anti-oxidant benefits? Try this recipe!

96. Honey Soy Salmon

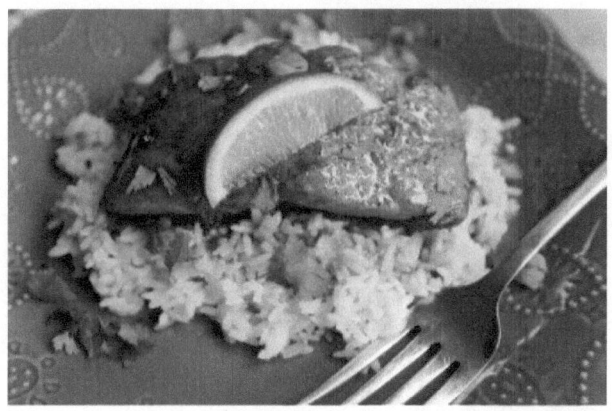

The Honey Soy Salmon is a really simple recipe that gives a real touch of sweetness without breaking its natural pleasing flavor.

Ingredients

- 1/5 Oz salmon fillet
- 1/2 Tablespoon soy sauce
- 1/2 tablespoon honey
- Pepper
- Salt

Method

1. Pre-heat the broiler. Combine soy sauce with honey.

2. Season salmon fillet with pepper and salt and broil for 5 minutes.

3. Drizzle with honey soy sauce. Broil for another 5 minutes. Serve with microwaveable rice.

Tips/Notes

Salmon fillet is a rich source of polyunsaturated and heart healthy fats.

97. Spicy Veggies

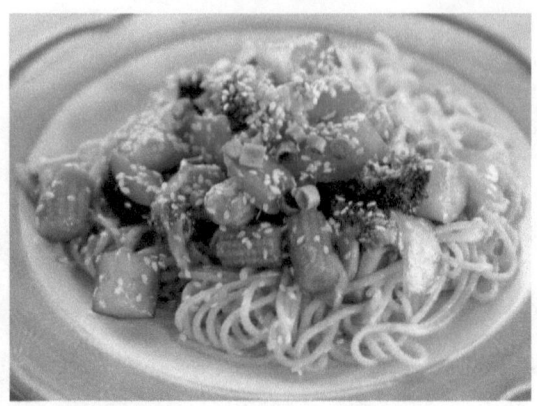

Hungry and want a meal that is truly fulfilling? Here is the spicy veggies recipe you've been looking for!

Ingredients

- 1/4 can drained and rinsed black beans
- 1/4 can drained and diced tomatoes
- 1/2 zucchini (diced)
- 1/4 cup diced okra
- Salt
- Hot sauce

Method

1. Combine drained diced tomatoes, drained and rinsed beans, diced okra and diced zucchini in a large skillet.

2. Cook for 10 minutes, or until cooked through. Stir in your preferred hot sauce. Add salt to taste.

Tips/Notes

Okra also known as gumbo pods are incredibly rich in health benefiting compounds like vitamin K, pyridoxine and anti-oxidants.

98. Springtime Stir-Fry

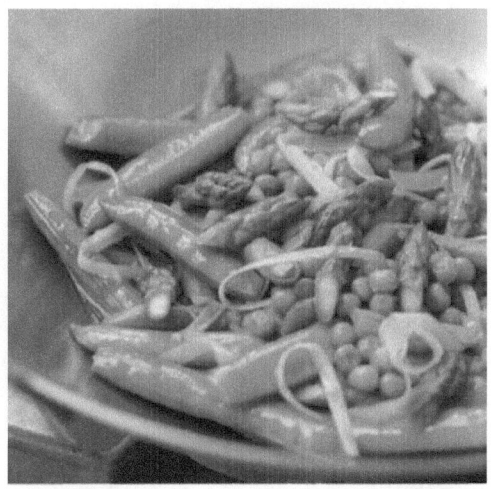

Do not omit canola oil—it adds just the true flavor component.

Ingredients

- 5 asparagus spears
- 5 asparagus spears
- 1/2 cup broccoli florets
- 1/4 cup (shelled) fava beans
- 2 tablespoons canola oil
- 1/2 tablespoon grated ginger
- 1 chopped scallion
- Rice (optional)

Method

1. Combine broccoli florets, snow peas, and fava beans in a pan coated with cooking spray.

2. Heat over medium heat and cook for 5 minutes. Heat grated ginger with canola oil and chopped scallion.

3. Toss with cooking veggies and cook for 4 more minutes. Serve with rice (optional).

Tips/Notes

Canola oil is one of the best oils for a healthy heart.

99. Spicy Shrimp Stir-Fry

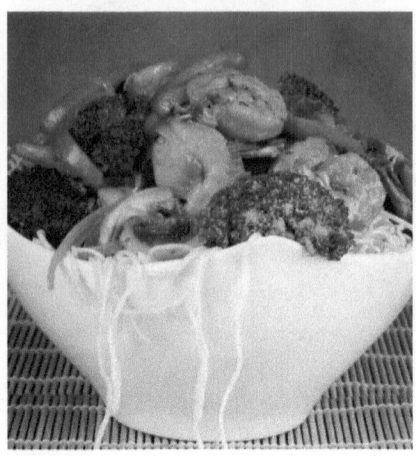

I have met stir-fries, at home or out at a restaurant but this one is different and you want to prepare it as soon as you get home!

Ingredients

- 1/4 lb. shelled and de-veined shrimp
- 1/4 cup corn kernels
- 1/2 cup thinly sliced squash and zucchini
- 1/2 red bell pepper (sliced)
- 1/4 onion (sliced)
- 1/8 tablespoon crushed red pepper
- 1 tablespoon canola oil

Method

1. Heat canola oil over medium heat. Add onion and crushed pepper and cook for 5 minutes.

2. Add zucchini, corn kernels, red bell pepper and thinly sliced squash.

3. Cook for 5 minutes and add shelled de-veined shrimp. Cook for 3 more.

Tips/Notes

Zucchini helps you attain your weight loss goals in a healthy style!

100. Turkey Frittata

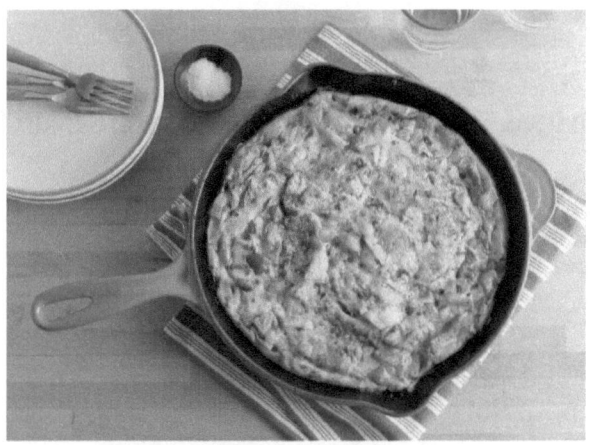

Bring your month of high flavored, tasty, delicious recipes to an end with this all-star, easy to follow Turkey Frittata recipe!

Ingredients

- 1/8 cup milk
- 1/2 tablespoon olive oil
- 2 eggs
- 1/8 cup grated onion
- Pepper
- A pinch of salt
- 1/2 tablespoon curry powder
- 1/4 lb. ground turkey

Method

1. Pre-heat the oven to 400 degrees. Heat olive oil over high heat in a small ovenproof pan. Add curry powder, ground turkey and grated onion. Cook until the turkey is no longer pink (about 5 minutes).

2. Meanwhile, beat together cup milk, eggs and a pinch of salt and pepper.

3. Add the egg mixture to the saucepan and lower the heat to medium-high. Cook until eggs begin to set. Transfer to the oven and cook until eggs set (about 5 minutes).

Tips/Notes

Did I mention that turkey has proven to aid in dealing with gout, high cholesterol and diabetes, tiredness and sleepiness?

101. Grilled Shrilled Skewers Over White Bean Salad

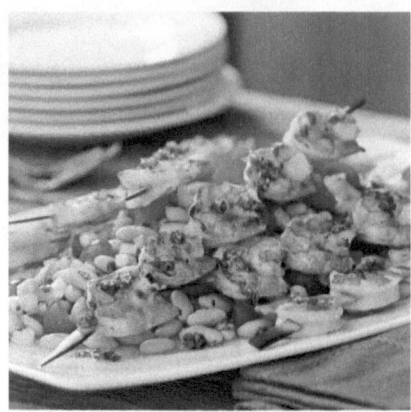

The two main ingredients of this dish; the grilled shrimp and the fresh bean salad go hand in hand and therefore, taste like heaven. The healthy nature of this barbeque dish is due to the fact that it contains fresh herbs and shrimps; the contents heavily recommended by dieticians and nutritionists.

Ingredients

- 1/3 cup lemon juice
- 3 tablespoons olive oil
- 2 tablespoons fresh minced oregano
- 2 tablespoons fresh minced chives
- 24 peeled and deveined raw shrimps
- 12 cherry tomatoes
- 1 teaspoon ground pepper
- 1/2 teaspoon salt
- 30-ounce cannellini beans

Method

1. Mix the lemon juice, olive oil, chives, oregano, salt and pepper in a bowl. Add beans and tomatoes to the paste and toss well. Heat the

grill to a medium high temperature to provide the optimum conditions.

2. Oil the skewers and stick the shrimps onto six of them and prepare them to be cooked. Make sure that you turn the skewers every four minutes so that the shrimps do not get burnt and they are cooked properly. Dress the shrimps in the end and serve them with the bean salad.

Tips/Notes

The lemon juice which has been used in this recipe has numerous advantages. The fact that it is slightly acidic in nature helps to break down the food in your stomach which aids in the effective and quick digestion.

102. Classic Hamburger

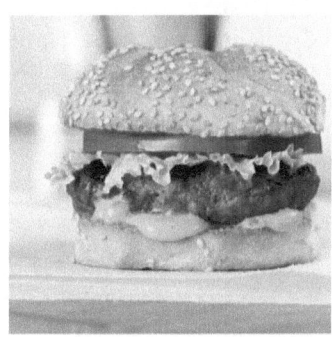

Who doesn't love burgers? Nobody! But if you are on a diet, trying to avoid all the high-calorie stuff, you are advised to stay away from them.

Classic Hamburger is here to rescue you as the lettuce leaves and onions are incredibly good for your health and allow you to consume your favorite hamburgers without any guilt.

Ingredients

- 1 tablespoon canola oil
- 1 medium sized onion
- 4 lettuce leaves
- 4 slices of tomato
- 2 tablespoons low fat mayonnaise

- 2 tablespoons tomato ketchup
- 1-pound ground beef
- 1 teaspoon white vinegar
- 2 tablespoons steak sauce
- 4 sesame seed buns
- 2 teaspoons pickle relish
- 1/2 teaspoon ground pepper

Method

1. Heat the grill to medium high temperature. Take the onion, oil and 1 tablespoon ketchup in a saucepan and heat at a medium high temperature until the onion acquires a brown color.

2. Lower the temperature to medium low and continue heating for another five minutes. Now combine mayonnaise, vinegar, relish and remaining ketchup in another bowl.

3. Meanwhile, add the beef, steak sauce and pepper to the already roasted onion and divide it to form four patties. Now toast the buns on the oiled grill and turn them once to avoid overheating. Assemble the burger on the grill and serve them with lettuce leaves, slices of tomato and tomato ketchup.

Tips/Notes

Most of the calories contained in burgers which is damaging for your health come from the mayonnaise. Using low fat mayonnaise instead can help contain this problem.

103. Green Chili Bison Burger

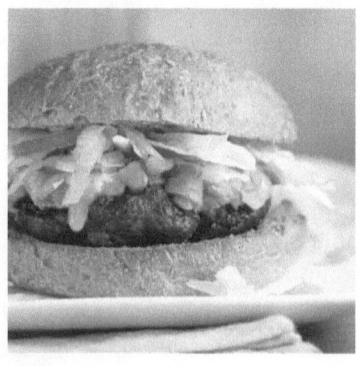

Continuing with the burgers, we have another tempting recipe for you which will turn the fortunes of the burger lovers who are currently watching their weight.

This is a South American dish whose main components are Bison meat and green chili which are grilled in such a way that it becomes a must-try for you.

Ingredients

- Quarter cup sliced red onion
- One-pound ground bison
- 8 ounces of green chili
- Half a cup of shredded cheese
- Quarter teaspoon salt
- Quarter teaspoon ground pepper
- 4 hamburger buns
- 1 cup sliced lettuce

Method

1. Heat the grill to a medium high temperature range and put the onions in a bowl filled with water and cover it for some time. Place the bison, chili, shredded cheese, salt and ground pepper in a separate bowl and mix the contents.

2. Form the mixture into 4 patties. Oil the grill and place the bison, cheese, chili combination on it and cook it at a medium high temperature. Turn the patties one by one and give each side about five minutes on the grill.

3. Put the remaining chili and cheese on the burger and heat it till the cheese melts. Assemble the patties on the buns and serve the burgers with the lettuce leaves and onion.

Tips/Notes

Bison burgers have less fat, cholesterol and fat than the average hamburgers due to which they are considered 'safe' to eat by most nutritionists.

104. Grilled Fish Tacos

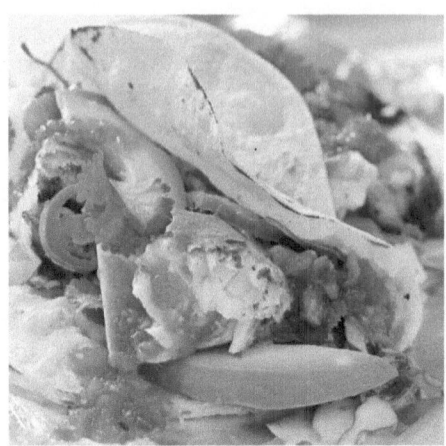

Instead of deep frying fish for making tacos which are have high fat and cholesterol content, we grill it and reduce the calorie level to a very safe amount. In this dish, it is made sure that the fillets are not too thick so that they take less time to cook and are heated equally on all sides.

Ingredients

- 2 tablespoons lime juice
- 2 tablespoons olive oil
- 4 teaspoons chili powder
- 1 teaspoon salt
- 1 teaspoon garlic powder
- 1 teaspoon onion powder
- Half teaspoon ground pepper
- 2 pounds Pacific halibut
- Quarter cup low fat sour cream
- Quarter cup low fat mayonnaise

Method

1. Heat the grill to a medium high temperature. Mix the fish with lime juice, olive oil, chili powder, garlic powder, onion powder, salt and pepper in a bowl and let it be for up to 30 minutes to allow the fish to catch the flavor.

2. To make coleslaw, mix the low-fat cream, low fat mayonnaise, salt, ground pepper, lime juice and sugar and refrigerate it until the tacos are completely cooked.

3. Now oil the grill and put the marinated fish on it and change the sides of the fish every five minutes to ensure balanced cooking. At the end, divide the fish into medium sized pieces and serve with coleslaw.

Tips/Notes

Taco is a traditional Mexican dish which has been eaten by the natives of Mexico since before the arrival of the Europeans in South America.

105. Grilled Chicken with A Touch of Chili and Lime

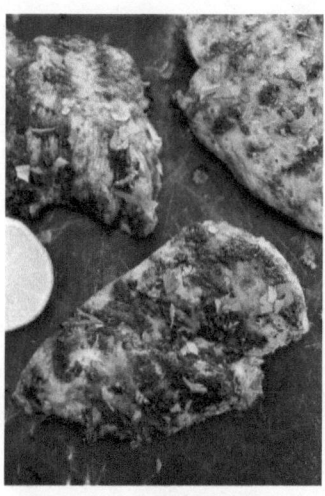

This recipe is cooked by using the butterflying technique which has become very popular over the last few decades. In this method, the chicken is grilled over direct heat at first and is then cooked over indirect heat. This aids in roasting the meat equally on the outside as well as the inside.

Ingredients

- 3 tablespoons chili powder
- 2 tablespoons lime zest
- 2 tablespoons olive oil
- 1 teaspoon oregano
- 1 tablespoon crushed garlic
- Three tablespoons lime juice
- One and a half teaspoon salt
- One teaspoon ground pepper
- 3½ to 4 pounds chicken

Method

1. Mix chili powder, lime zest, olive oil, oregano, garlic, lime juice, salt and pepper in a bowl to form a paste. Now cut the chicken in such a way that its backbone is completely removed and all the pieces obtained are perfectly symmetric.

2. Marinate the chicken with the wet sauce prepared in the first step. Place a bowl or a dish over the chicken and refrigerate for at least 24 hours.

3. Heat half the grill to a medium high temperature and place the marinated chicken pieces on the grill. Turn the pieces every five minutes to ensure balanced cooking. When the pieces turn brown, remove them and put them in a platter. Serve the grilled chicken with tomato ketchup, onions and tomato slices.

Tips/Notes

Grilled chicken with chili and lime serves you with 25 percent of your daily vitamin A requirement. This vitamin is essential for the normal functioning of eyes, teeth, bone metabolism and immunity.

106. Steak, Potato Kebabs and Cilantro Sauce

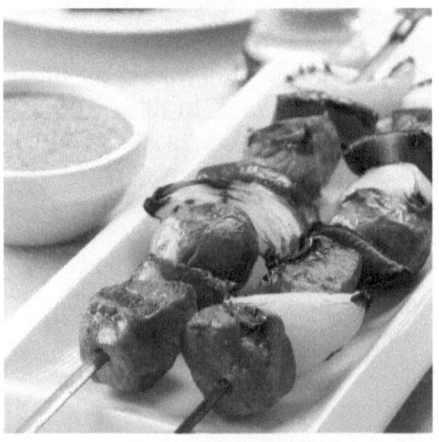

To add to the nutritional value of a well-cooked steak, it is served with potatoes, onions, salads and a delicious cilantro sauce in this recipe. The potatoes are precooked in a microwave oven and then grilled with the steak so that both the parts of the meal are readied at the exact same time.

Ingredients

- Half a cup of crushed cilantro leaves
- 2 tablespoons vinegar
- 2 tablespoons low fat sour cream
- 1 teaspoons chili powder
- Half teaspoon salt
- 8 small red potatoes
- A quarter pound strip steak
- 1 teaspoon olive oil
- One large sweet onion

Method

1. Take the cilantro leaves, vinegar, sour cream, chili powder and salt in a bowl, mix it and set it aside. Heat the grill to a medium high temperature range. Put the potatoes in a microwave and allow them to get soft on heating for about three minutes.

2. Take the potatoes, steak, pepper, salt and oil in another bowl and mix the contents well. Put the steak, potatoes and onions on the skewers and grill them for about five minutes.

3. Turn the skewers after every five minutes and make sure that the steak and potatoes are cooked evenly. Serve the dish with the sauce which was prepared in the first step.

Tips/Notes

This recipe is rich in zinc and fulfills more than 35 percent of the daily requirements. A deficiency of zinc in the human body can result in diseases related to liver, diabetes and other chronic illnesses.

107. Moroccan Shrimp with Spinach

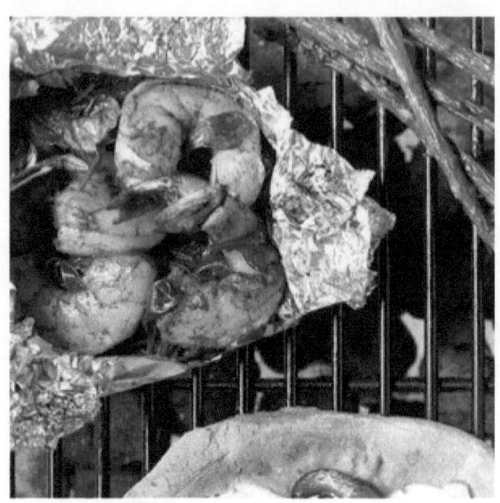

This African recipe has spinach as its primary ingredient and also contains the grilling of shrimp in a medium high temperature range in the cooking procedure. The preparation time for this dish is almost forty minutes and cooking time is not more than seven minutes which allows it to be grilled in just under an hour.

Ingredients

- Half teaspoon coriander
- Half teaspoon cumin
- Half teaspoon paprika
- Quarter teaspoon salt
- 1 Pound large deveined and peeled shrimp
- 10 ounces spinach
- 3 tablespoons olive oil

Method

1. First of all, mix the coriander, cumin, paprika and salt in a small bowl in a homogenous manner. Take the shrimp in another bowl and coat it in the mixture of the spices, allow it to rest for thirty minutes and refrigerate it.

2. Now, take spinach, oil and salt in another large bowl, mix it and place it evenly on a sheet of aluminum along with the shrimp. Bring the edges of the foil together and seal them so that the whole setting becomes airtight.

3. Now, put the aluminum sheets on the grill and start heating it. Allow the shrimp and spinach to be cooked for another five to seven minutes and wait until the shrimp becomes opaque. Serve the dish with sauces and tomato ketchup.

Tips/Notes

Aluminum foil grilling is a type of indirect grilling. This is done to prevent the meat and fire from coming into direct contact with each other. Indirect grilling is done in order to preserve the nutritional value of food and for stopping it from being overcooked.

108. Grilled Steak Served with Fresh Corn Salad

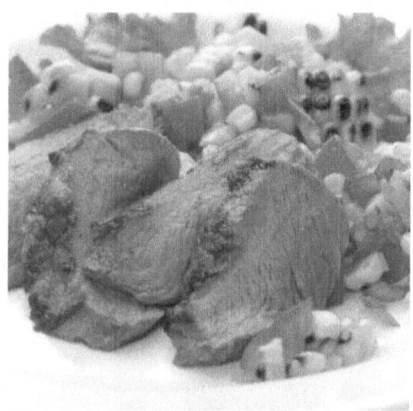

The key to having the perfect meal here is to prepare the ingredients of the salad beforehand. Then you can grill the steak and mix the salad to serve them both together while the steak is still fresh and juicy.

Ingredients

- 1 tablespoon garlic
- 3 teaspoons olive oil
- Half teaspoon salt
- 2 trimmed boneless strip pounds (1.25 pounds)
- 5 ears husked corn
- 2 chopped medium sized tomatoes
- 1 small red bell pepper
- 2 tablespoons basil
- 2 tablespoons vinegar

113

Method

1. Heat the grill to high temperature. Mix together garlic, some oil and a quarter teaspoon salt. Apply this blend on the sides of the steaks. Put the steak and corn on the grill for 2 to 4 minutes each side. Let the steak rest while the corn is cooked.

2. Keep cooking the corn; turn it to spread the heat all around the corn equally until some of the kernels are charred. This should take around 8 minutes. Now take it off and give it about 5 minutes so that they become cool enough to handle.

3. Use a knife to remove the kernels off of the ears of the corn. Mix the corn with tomatoes and pepper; and then stir it with basil, vinegar, salt and oil. Finish the steak by slicing them and serve them together with the salad.

Tips/Notes

Although it has been 500,000 years since meat has been grilled, it did not become very common until the middle of the 20th century.

109. Smoky Ham and Corn Salad

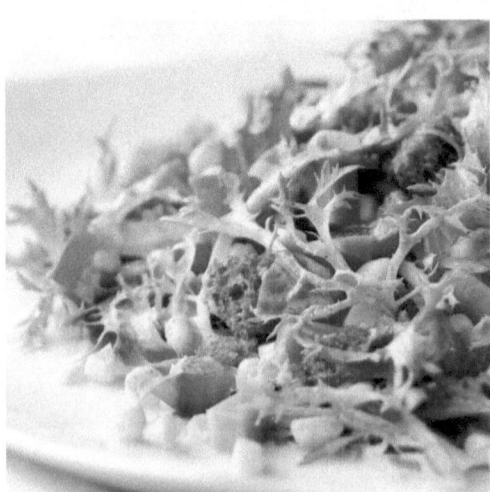

Fresh corn, chopped deli ham and crispy croutons are mixed with a smoky, rich dressing in this light summer salad. Best served with a crisp glass of sliced melon and rosé.

Ingredients

- A one-third cup of sour cream
- 2 tablespoons of vinegar
- A teaspoon of paprika
- One-quarter teaspoon of salt
- A medium sized tomato
- A cup of corn kernels; fresh
- A cup of whole grain croutons
- Three-fourth of a cup diced ham

Method

1. Firstly, whisk sour cream in a bowl. Then add some vinegar, paprika and salt in the bowl. Try to use a large one to ensure that all the ingredients mix together really well.

2. Now add salad greens to the mixture. Finally finish by adding the diced tomato, corn kernels, croutons and ham. Mix all the ingredients really well.

Tips/Notes

Ham is one of the oldest meats in human civilization. It is claimed that the French invented the treatment of pork to produce ham.

110. Grilled Steak with Pepper Relish

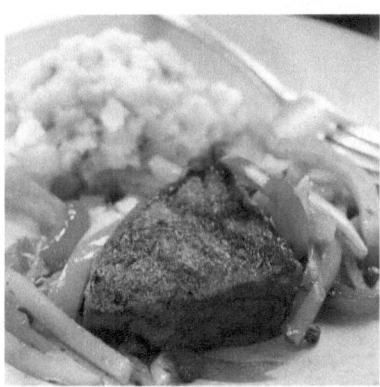

Bell peppers is mixed in vinaigrette and grilled in a foil at the same time as the steak is grilled. It is served with corn.

Ingredients

- 3 small sliced bell peppers
- 1 halved and sliced small onion
- 2 tablespoons of vinegar; preferably balsamic
- 1 tablespoon of olive oil
- 1 tablespoon of rinsed capers
- 1 tablespoon fresh thyme; freshly chopped or 1 teaspoon dried and divided thyme
- Half teaspoon salt
- Half teaspoon of ground pepper
- A pound of sirloin steak; preferably 1-1.25 inches thick. Cut into four portions
- A teaspoon of garlic powder

Method

1. Heat the grill to a medium level. Mix the peppers with oil, vinegar, capers, 2 of the teaspoons of fresh thyme and a quarter teaspoon of each pepper and salt in a bowl. Lay out the two and a half feet foil and put the mixture of pepper earlier made on one half. Now fold the foil and make sure that the foil is sealed properly so that the mixture does not leak during the grilling.

2. Now apply some garlic powder, quarter teaspoon of salt and pepper on each side of the steak. Oil the grill rack. You can do this by folding a paper towel, oiling it, holding it with tongs and rubbing it on the rack.

3. Now, place the packed foil and the steak on the grill. Grill the steak for 4 to 5 minutes per side. Grill the foil packet for 10 to 12 minutes during which time the vegetables should be tender. Now allow the steak to rest on the grill (no heat) for 5 minutes. Serve the juicy steak along with the peppers.

Tips/Notes

Grilling is perhaps the best method to cook meat because all the fat is melted away giving you just the healthy proteins.

111. Mojito-Rubbed Chicken with Grilled Pineapple

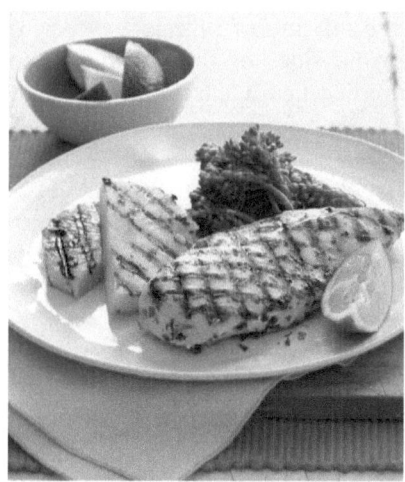

You can give the typical grilled chicken a twist with some added lime and mint!

Ingredients

- 4 chicken breast halves; skinless and boneless
- 2 limes
- 1 tablespoon of olive oil
- A medium sized pineapple
- 0.25 c. fresh mint leaves; loosely packed
- Pepper and salt

Method

1. Prepare the grill on medium. Use a meat mallet to beat the chicken to a flat half an inch thickness. Wrap the chicken between two plastic wrap sheets before pounding it. Use 1 lime to squeeze two tablespoons of juice and a teaspoon of peel. Then cut the other lime into four pieces. Set these aside for now. Combine oil, juice, peel and lime together in a bowl.

2. Now brush the pineapple softly on each of the two sides with the lime mixture earlier prepared. Set aside the remaining mixture.

3. Now place these slices of pineapple on the hot grill. Cook for 10 minutes. After the 10 minutes, both sides should turn brown. During the cooking, make sure that you turn it over once.

4. Now pull out the mixture of lime left earlier. Add some mint into it and apply it to the sides of the chicken. Season both sides of the chicken by sprinkling half a teaspoon of salt and a quarter teaspoon of ground pepper on both sides.

5. Now cook the chicken on a hot grill for about 5 minutes. The chicken should turn brown on both of the sides. It is served with wedges of lime and pineapple.

Tips/Notes

Back in 1980, about 10 percent of a chicken's weight was from breast meat. In 2007, the percentage of breast meat in a chicken's total meat was 21 percent.

112. Spiced Pork Tenderloins with Mango Salsa

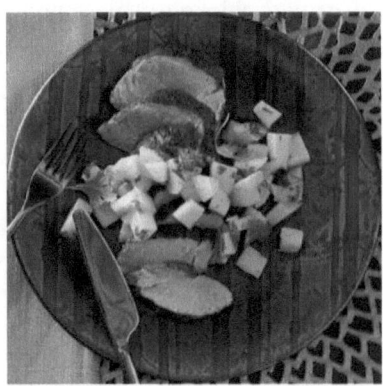

Add a delicious Mango Salsa to a dish as loved as Spiced Pork Tenderloins and you have the most exciting combination of dishes you can have.

Ingredients

- 2 mangoes; medium sized ripe
- 2 kiwifruits; medium sized
- 2 tablespoon vinegar
- 1 tablespoon fresh ginger; grated and peeled
- 1 tablespoon cilantro leaves
- 2 pork tenderloins
- 3 tablespoons of flour
- A teaspoon of salt
- A teaspoon of cumin; ground
- A teaspoon of coriander; ground

- Half teaspoon of cinnamon; ground
- Half teaspoon of ginger; ginger

Method

1. First, prepare the Mango Salsa. Mix mangoes, vinegar, cilantro, kiwifruit and ginger in a medium sized bowl. The aforementioned ingredients make about 4 cups. If it is not being served right after being prepared, cover and refrigerate it for up to 4 hours.

2. Preheat the grill for grilling over medium level heat. Cut the pork tenderloins in half lengthwise. Make sure that you do not cut all the way through the meat. Take plastic wrap sheets and place each one between two sheets. Use a meat mallet to pound the meat into flat quarter inch thickness.

3. Mix some flour, coriander, ground ginger, cinnamon, salt, cumin on paper. Now add the pork to this mixture to spice it up. Turn it over to ensure that the spice mixture sticks to the meat evenly on all sides.

4. Now put the spice mixture added pork on the preheated grill rack. Cook it until the meat loses its pink color and turns a light shade of brown. Turn over the pork once to cook it evenly on both sides. Serve the cooked pork with Mango Salsa.

Tips/Notes

Pork has more protein than chicken and is high in zinc, iron and B-vitamins.

113. Steak Sandwich with Grilled Onion

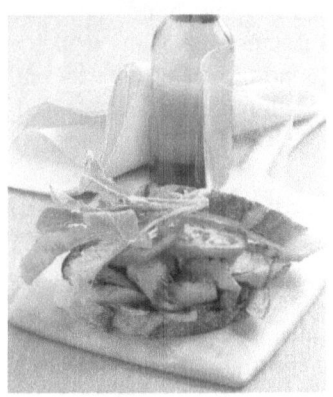

Treat yourself with a classy steak sandwich optimized by the presence of the crisp, grilled onion.

Ingredients

- A tablespoon of brown sugar
- A teaspoon of thyme leaves; fresh
- A beef steak
- A red onion, medium sized
- 8 slices of sourdough bread
- 2 ripe tomatoes; medium sized
- A bunch of arugula
- Quarter cup of soy sauce
- Quarter cup of vinegar; balsamic
- Quarter teaspoon of pepper; ground

Method

1. Use a plastic bag that is self-sealing to ensure that nothing leaks out. Pour mix soy sauce, pepper, thyme, vinegar and sugar into this plastic bag. Marinade steak by adding steak into this mixture. Turn it over to ensure even application. Now place the bag on a plate and let it rest for about fifteen minutes. Turn it over a few times.

2. Now preheat the grill to medium heat. To help in the handling, insert a metal skewer through the slices of the onion and set it aside.

3. Now remove the steak from the marinade and pour the marinade into a pan. Boil the marinade for two minutes by heating it over high heat.

4. Now put the slices of onion and the steak on the grill for around twelve to fifteen minutes. Cover the grill for better heating. When the onions turn brown and the meat loses its pink color, it is done. During the heating, keep applying the marinade and keep turning it over from time to time to make sure that it is heated evenly on both sides.

5. Once done, move the steak from the grill and take it to the cutting board. Now divide the cooked onion into rings.

6. Finally, slice the steak across its grain. Take four slices of bread and place the sliced steak and rings of onion on it. If there are any meat juices left over on the cutting board, pour them over the steak and the

onion. Finish the dressing with tomatoes, arugula and the other four bread slices.

Tips/Notes

As far as grill foods are concerned, burgers (85 percent) and steak (80 percent) are the most popular dishes.

114. Juicy Rosemary Chicken Skewer Kabobs

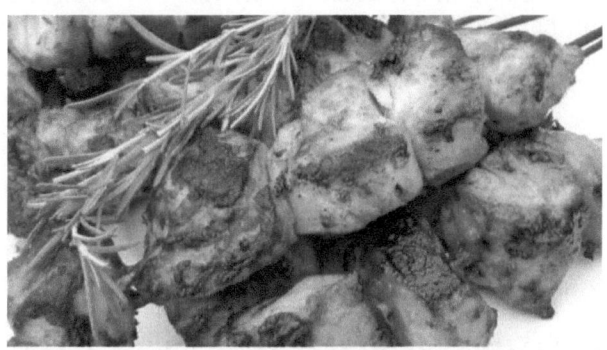

This delicious Kabob recipe is really delicious and extremely tender, with the kabobs almost melting on your tongue. Even the pickiest eater won't be able to stay away from it!

Ingredients

- 1 cup extra virgin olive oil
- 1 cup ranch dressing
- 6 tablespoons Worcestershire sauce
- 2 tablespoons fresh rosemary, minced
- 4 teaspoons salt
- 2 teaspoons fresh lemon juice
- 2 teaspoons white vinegar
- 1/2 teaspoon ground black pepper, or to taste
- 2 tablespoons white sugar, or to taste
- 10 boneless and skinless chicken breast halves, cubed

Method

1. Place the ranch dressing, olive oil, rosemary, Worcestershire sauce, lemon juice, salt, pepper, white vinegar and sugar in a medium sized bowl and give it a stir. Set the bowl aside for about 5 to 7 minutes, so

that the sugar easily dissolves. Place the boneless chicken breast cubes in the bowl with the marinade and toss to quote. Cover using a cling wrap and place in the refrigerator for about 30 minutes.

2. Turn the grill on a medium-high heat and let it preheat while the chicken marinates. Thread the marinated chicken cubes onto greased skewers and discard the remaining marinade.

3. Spray the grill with some cooking spray. Place the prepared skewers on the greased grill and cook the skewers for about 10 to 12 minutes or until the center of the chicken is no longer pink. Serve hot with a side of your favorite condiment!

Tips/Notes

It is common knowledge that marinating meats before cooking ensures that the meat cooks easily. But, if you are cooking smaller pieces of meat, do not marinate the meat for too long, or else the meat will get over tender and fall apart on the grill.

115. Grilled Garlic and Pepper Steak with A Caprese Salad

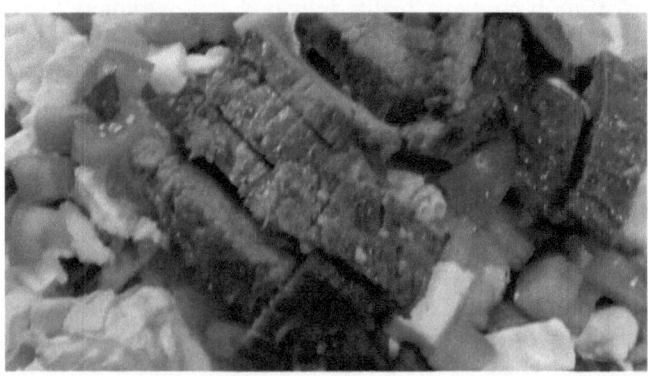

This delicious garlic and pepper flavored steak tastes delicious with a side of the delicious and healthy salad makes for a healthy and nutritious meal. This recipe is for 8 portions.

Ingredients

- 4 tomatoes, cut into cubes
- 8 ounces fresh mozzarella, chopped into 1-inch cubes
- 1/2 cup fresh basil, roughly chopped
- 2 cloves of garlic, minced (you may add more for added flavor)

- 2 tablespoons extra virgin olive oil
- 2 pounds lean flank steak
- 2 cloves of garlic, minced
- 2 tablespoons extra virgin olive oil
- Salt, to taste
- freshly ground black pepper, to taste
- 1 ½ cup lettuce
- 1/4 cup balsamic vinegar, or to taste
- Extra virgin olive oil, to taste

Method

1. In a large mixing bowl, combine together the basil, mozzarella cheese, 2 minced garlic cloves and the 2 tablespoons of extra virgin olive oil and toss well to coat. Cover the bowl using a cling wrap and place in the refrigerator.

2. Turn the grill up to medium-high heat and preheat it for a few minutes. Spray the grill with some cooking oil.

3. Take a large re-sealable bag and place the 2 minced garlic cloves, 2 tablespoons extra virgin olive oil, pepper and salt in it. Place the steak in the bag and seal the bag. Shake the bag well to evenly distribute the marinade mixture on the steak.

4. Place the steak on the greased grill and cook them to your taste. For a medium steak cook the steak for about 5 minutes on each side. A kitchen thermometer inserted in the center of the steak should read 140 degrees Fahrenheit (about 60 degrees Celsius). Once the steak is taken off the grill, let the steak sit out for about 5 minutes and then slice it against the grain.

5. Remove the salad from the refrigerator and divide the lettuce among 8 serving plates. Spoon the balsamic vinegar and olive oil onto the serving plates. Place about 1/8 of the grilled steak on the lettuce and top with about 1/8 of the prepared salad on the steak.

Did you know?

When you accompany your meal with a refreshing salad, it adds to the nutritional and satiating value of your meal.

116. Quick and Easy Italian Grilled Chicken

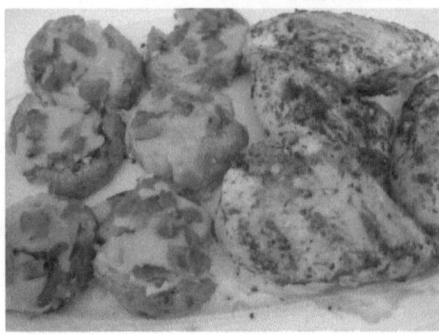

This is the quickest and easiest way to marinade and cook chicken, ideal for new cooks.

Ingredients

- 8 boneless and skinless chicken breast halves
- 2 teaspoons garlic powder
- 4 cups Italian-style salad dressing of your choice
- 2 teaspoons salt

Method

1. Combine the garlic powder and salad dressing in a medium sized bowl. Add in the salt and mix well. Place the chicken breast halves in this mix and keep turning them to coat well. Cover the bowl using a cling wrap and place in the refrigerator for about 4 hours. It is preferable to marinate overnight for best results!

2. Turn the grill up to the highest heat and let the grill preheat. Spray the grill with some cooking spray. Drain the excess marinade from the chicken and place the breast halves on the greased grill.

3. Grill the chicken breasts for about 8 minutes on each side. Remove from grill and let it rest for a few minutes, before slicing it against the grain. Serve hot with a side of your favorite condiment.

Tips/Notes

The garlic powder used in this recipe has all the properties of fresh garlic and helps with the reduction of the cholesterol levels in the body.

117. Paprika Shrimp with Lemon Aioli

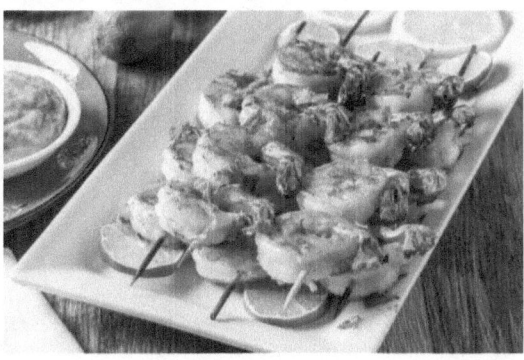

Though the list of ingredients in this recipe may make the dish seem to be extremely bland and tasteless, but the cured lemons have an extremely intense flavor that adds to the dish. But, if you would like some extra flavor in the dish, add some hot pepper or garlic in it.

Ingredients

- 4 slices of cured lemon
- 1 cup mayonnaise
- 2 tablespoons fresh tarragon, minced
- 2 teaspoons lemon juice
- 2 pounds extra-large shrimp, peeled and deveined
- 4 teaspoons extra virgin olive oil
- 2 teaspoons smoked paprika
- 1 teaspoon kosher salt

Method

1. Pour some cold water in a small bowl and soak the cured lemons in it for about 10 minutes, in order to get rid of the curing brine. Place the drained lemons on an absorbent towel to dry. Mince the lemon finely.

2. In a small mixing bowl combine the mayonnaise, lemon juice, tarragon and minced lemon together. Cover the bowl using a cling wrap and refrigerate until chilled. If you do not have too long, refrigerate for at least 15 minutes.

3. Turn up your grill to high heat and let it preheat for at least 10 minutes. Spray some cooking spray on the grill to grease it.

4. Place the peeled and deveined shrimp in a bowl and pour the extra virgin olive oil over them. Lightly sprinkle the kosher salt and smoked paprika on the shrimp and mix well until the shrimp are well coated.

5. Place the marinated shrimp on the greased and preheated grill and cook for about 2 minutes on each side or until they get a bright pink tinge and the meat loses its transparency. Serve hot with the prepared lemon aioli.

Tips/Notes

Lemons aid in restoring the natural pH levels in the body and aid in the detoxification of the digestive system. Lemons also aid in smooth digestion and prevent the occurrence of constipation in the body.

118. Chicken Souvlaki with a delicious Tzatziki Sauce

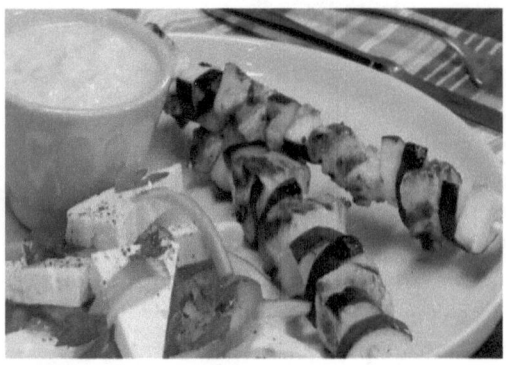

Souvlaki is a traditional Greek dish which contains grilled vegetables and meats and is usually served with a dipping sauce. These delicious kabobs have a delicious Greek flavor and the marinade can also be used to flavor other meats like beef and pork too!

Ingredients

- 1/2 cup extra virgin olive oil
- 1/4 cup lemon juice
- 4 cloves of garlic, crushed
- 2 teaspoons dried oregano
- 1 teaspoon salt
- 3 pounds chicken breast halves, boneless and skinless, chopped into small pieces

For the Sauce

- 1 ½ cups Greek-style yogurt, unflavored
- 1 cucumber, peeled, seeds removed and grated
- 2 tablespoons extra virgin olive oil
- 4 teaspoons white vinegar
- 2 cloves of garlic, minced
- 2 pinches of salt
- 12 wooden skewers, or as you need

Method

1. Pour the ½ cup extra virgin olive oil into a re-sealable bag. Add in the 4 minced garlic cloves, 1 teaspoon salt and the 2 teaspoons of dried oregano. Place the chicken in the bag, seal it and slowly shake it up to ensure that the chicken is well coated with the marinade. Place the bag in the refrigerator and let the chicken marinate for about 3 to 4 hours.

2. While the chicken marinates, prepare the dipping sauce. Pour the yogurt in to a small mixing bowl. Add in the grated cucumber, the 2 tablespoons extra virgin olive oil, white vinegar, the 2 cloves of minced garlic and the salt to it. Mix well and place the prepared tzatziki sauce in the refrigerator. Chill for at least 3 hours.

3. Turn up your grill on a medium high flame and let it preheat for a few minutes. Grease the grill with some cooking spray. Place the skewers in some warm water and let them soak for 15 to 20 minutes.

4. Remove the marinated pieces of chicken and thread them onto the prepared skewers. Drain and discard the leftover marinade.

5. Place the prepared skewers on the greased and preheated grill. Keep turning the skewers frequently so that the chicken is evenly browned from all sides. It should take about 10 minutes. Serve hot with the prepared tzatziki sauce.

Tips/Notes

The tzatziki is a delicious Greek dipping sauce and it goes amazingly well with all kinds of meat preparations. The traditional dipping sauce usually uses yoghurt made using the milk from goats and sheep.

119. Sweet and Spicy Grilled Pork Tenderloin

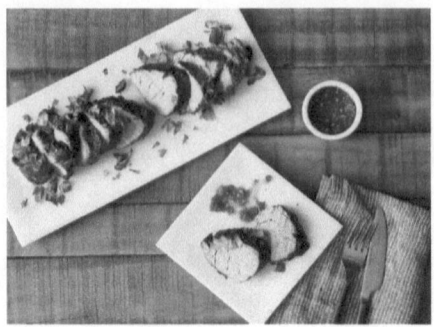

This delicious rub gives the pork tenderloins a sweet and spicy flavor. Just marinate the tenderloins and leave them for a few minutes. Grill and you are good to go!

Ingredients

- 2 teaspoons onion powder
- 2 teaspoons garlic powder
- 6 tablespoons chipotle chili powder
- 1 tablespoon salt
- 1/2 cup brown sugar
- 4 pork tenderloins, each about ¾ pound

Method

1. Turn up your grill to a medium high flame and coat it with some cooking spray. Take a large re-sealable bag and add the garlic powder, onion powder, salt, brown sugar and chipotle chili powder to it. Place the tenderloins in the bag with the marinade and shake the bag to evenly coat the tenderloin with the marinade. Place the bag in the refrigerator for about 20 minutes.

2. Place the pork tenderloins on the greased grill and cook for about 20 to 25 minutes. Make sure to turn over the tenderloins every 7 minutes.

3. Once done, remove the tenderloins from the grill and let them rest for about 10 minutes before slicing it. Serve hot.

Tips/Notes

If you want to lose weight the consumption of pork tenderloin is way better than the consumption of a chicken breast.

120. Bacon Stuffed Zucchini Boats

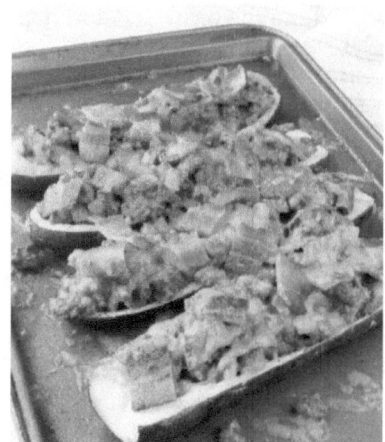

Stuffed grilled zucchini that makes a delicious appetizer or a light meal!

Ingredients

- 4 medium zucchini
- 2 slices white bread, cut into bite sizes
- 1/2 cup bacon, crumbled
- 2 tablespoons black olives, minced finely
- 2 jalapeno peppers, minced
- 6 tablespoons green chili peppers, diced
- 1/2 cup onion, minced
- 1/2 cup tomato, chopped
- 3/4 cup Cheddar cheese, shredded
- 2 pinches dried basil
- salt to taste
- ground black pepper to taste

Method

1. Prepare the grill in order to indirectly heat the zucchini boats. Pour enough water to cover the zucchini in a pot. Heat the pot until the water is boiling and let the zucchini cook for another 5 minutes.

2. Drain the zucchini and cool completely before cutting them lengthwise in halves. Using a small spoon, spoon out the flesh of the zucchini and chop the pulp.

3. Combine the prepared zucchini pulp, crumbled bacon, bread pieces, jalapenos, olives, onions, green chili peppers, Cheddar cheese and tomato in a bowl. Add in the basil, salt and pepper.

4. Spoon the prepared filling mix into the scooped-out zucchini halves. Cover the zucchini halves with some foil to seal them.

5. Place the prepared zucchini boats on the prepared grill and cook them for about 20 minutes or until the zucchini is tender to touch. Serve hot.

Tips/Notes

Zucchini has no saturated fats in it. It is an extremely good source of dietary fibers and helps prevent the cancer of the colon.

121. Rosemary Stuffed, Bacon Wrapped Chicken

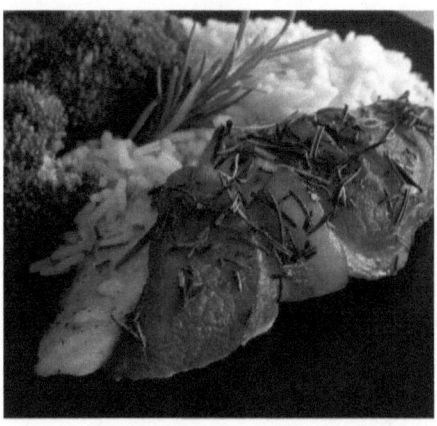

This recipe is ideal for the days when you are in no mood to do a lot of prep. Grill it up and serve with a side of some rice and grilled veggies.

Ingredients

- 8 teaspoons garlic powder
- 8 chicken breast halves, skinless and boneless
- Salt, to taste
- Pepper, to taste
- 8 sprigs fresh rosemary
- 8 thick slices bacon

Method

1. Turn up your grill on a medium high flame and lightly spray the grill with some cooking spray.

2. Dust a teaspoon of garlic powder on a single chicken breast. Sprinkle salt and pepper and place a rosemary sprig on it. Take the slice of bacon and wrap it around the chicken breast in order to secure the rosemary sprig in place. Secure the bacon in place using a toothpick.

3. Place the prepared chicken breast on the prepared grill and cook until the chicken is no longer pink in the center. This will take about 8 minutes per side. Remove the toothpicks and serve hot!

Tips/Notes

Rosemary is an extremely good source of anti-inflammatory compounds and anti-oxidants that help with the immune system of the body and also aids in healthy digestion.

122. Sweet n Spicy Grilled Pineapple Rings

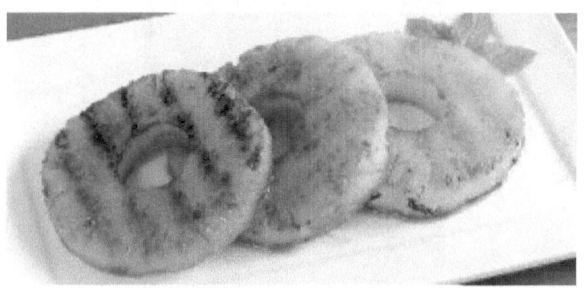

If you are a sucker for sweet and spicy, this will be your favorite dish in no time. Hot sauce cuts into the sweetness of the pineapple, giving it a delicious flavor that will leave you begging for more!

Ingredients

- 2 fresh pineapples, peeled, cored and cut into rings
- 1/2 teaspoon honey
- 6 tablespoons melted butter
- ¼ teaspoon hot pepper sauce
- salt to taste

Method

1. In a large re-sealable bag place the pineapple rings. Pour in the honey, hot pepper sauce, butter and salt and seal the bag. Shake the bag until the pineapple is well coated with the marinade. Leave it to marinate overnight.

2. Turn up your grill to the highest heat and lightly spray the grill with some cooking spray.

3. Place the prepared pineapple pieces on the grill and cook for 3 minutes per side or until lightly tender. Serve immediately.

Tips/Notes

The acidic and stinging taste you get when you consume a pineapple is due to the presence of the Bromelaine enzyme in it. The Bromelaine enzyme breaks down protein; so, when you eat the pineapple, it eats you!

123. Hamburgers Topped with Mushrooms and Swiss Cheese

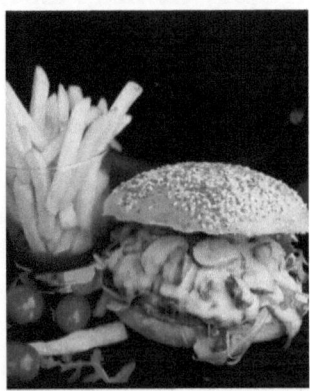

If you are tired of eating the regular ordinary hamburger, this recipe is your ticket to something mind-blowingly fantastic!

Ingredients

- 3/4-pound lean ground beef
- 1/4 teaspoon seasoned meat tenderizer
- Salt, to taste
- Pepper, to taste
- 1 teaspoon butter

- 1 (4 ounce) can sliced mushrooms, drained
- 1 tablespoon soy sauce
- 3 slices Swiss cheese
- 3 hamburger buns

Method

1. Turn on the grill to medium high heat and spray it with some cooking spray. Divide the lean ground beef into 3 parts and shape into patties. Sprinkle the salt, pepper and meat tenderizer on them and keep aside.

2. Place the butter in a skillet and heat over a medium flame until it has melted. Add in the drained mushrooms and the soy sauce and toss well until the mushrooms are browned. Take off heat but keep warm.

3. Place the prepared patties on the grill and cook for about 8 minutes on each side. Distribute the prepared mushrooms on the patties and place one slice of cheese on each patty. Cover the grill and cook for one minute or until the cheese melts. Remove from grill, place on the hamburger buns and serve hot!

Tips/Notes

The 28th of May every year is celebrated as National Hamburger Day!

124. Tandoori Chicken Thighs

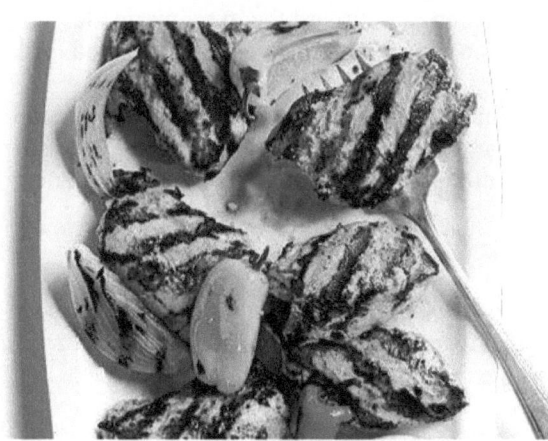

With the freshness of yogurt, this spicy dish will sure leave you yearning for more!

Ingredients

- ¾ cup plain yogurt
- 1 teaspoon kosher salt
- 1/2 teaspoon black pepper corns
- 1/4 teaspoon cloves, ground
- 1 tablespoon ginger, freshly grated
- 1-1/2 cloves garlic, minced
- 2 teaspoons paprika
- 1 teaspoon cumin, ground
- 1 teaspoon cinnamon, ground
- 1 teaspoon coriander seeds, ground
- 8 chicken thighs
- Olive oil spray

Method

1. Combine the yogurt, pepper corns, kosher salt, ground cloves and grated ginger and mix well. Add in the cinnamon, paprika, coriander seeds, garlic and cumin to it. Keep aside.

2. Rinse the chicken and pat dry. Take a large re-sealable bag and place the chicken in it. Add the prepared yoghurt mix to it and seal the bag. Shake a few times to distribute the marinade and refrigerate overnight.

3. Turn up the grill to medium and let it preheat. Drain the marinade from the chicken and discard the extra marinade. Spray some olive oil on the chicken pieces and place on the preheated grill.

4. Cook the chicken for 2 minutes on each side. Arrange the grill so that the chicken can get indirect heat. Keep cooking the chicken for another 40 minutes. Serve hot with some yogurt and cucumber dip.

Tips/Notes

The tandoor traditionally is an oven made of clay, used to grill meats and bake breads. The dishes made in a traditional tandoor have a distinct flavor that they get from being cooked in the clay oven.

125. Honey Flavored Grilled Shrimp

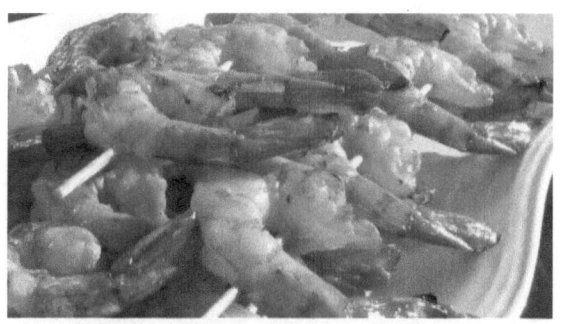

This recipe is ideal for the days when you want to make a quick and delicious dish without putting in hours of work!

Ingredients

- 2 pounds medium sized shrimp, peeled and deveined
- 1 cup chili-garlic sauce
- 1 cup honey
- 12 bamboo skewers, soaked in water for 20 minutes

Method

1. Turn the grill up on a medium high heat and lightly spray cooking spray on the grill. Combine the honey and chili-garlic sauce in a small bowl.

2. Skewer the shrimp on the soaked bamboo skewers, with the skewer going through the head and coming out through the tail side.

3. Place the skewers on the greased grill and grill the shrimp, while constantly basting it with the prepared sauce mix. Keep grilling until the shrimps until they are firm and get a pink tinge to them. This will take about 10 minutes. Serve hot!

Tips/Notes

Honey is one of the only foods in the world that doesn't spoil; in fact, archaeologists have found jars of honey in ancient Egyptian tombs and this honey is still edible!

126. Spicy Asian Pork Skewers

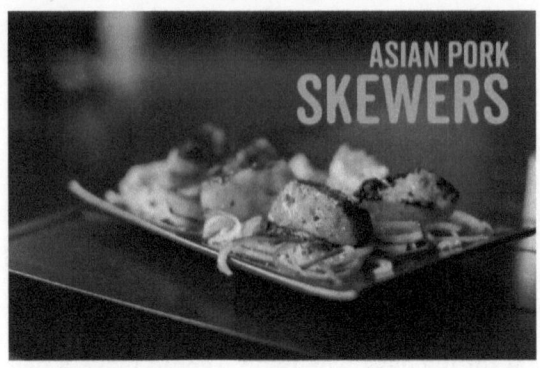

These kabobs are quick to prepare, with the Teriyaki sauce giving them an intense Asian flavor.

Ingredients

- 4 tablespoons teriyaki sauce
- 2 tablespoons red wine vinegar
- 2 tablespoons vegetable oil
- 2 teaspoons brown sugar
- 1 teaspoon red pepper flakes
- 1-1/2 pounds pork tenderloin, cut into 1-inch cubes

Method

1. Combine the teriyaki sauce, vegetable oil, pepper flakes, red wine vinegar and brown sugar in a medium sized bowl. Add the cubed pork tenderloin and toss well, until coated. Marinate overnight or a minimum of 30 – 45 minutes.

2. Turn up your grill to high and preheat. Lightly spray cooking oil on the grill.

3. Thread the marinated pork cubes on to skewers and place on the grill. Cook for about 12 minutes, constantly rotating the skewers and basting them with the leftover marinade. Serve hot!

Tips/Notes

Teriyaki is actually a technique used in Japanese cooking. It consists of grilling or broiling meats that are coated with a mixture of mirin, soy sauce and sugar.

127. Sweet and Savory Salmon on The Grill

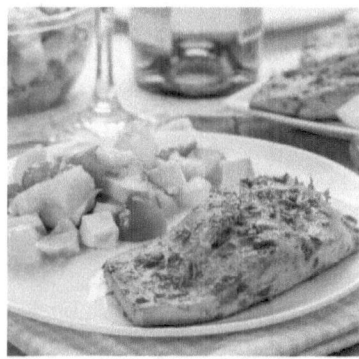

The intense flavor of this dish consists of a perfect balance between the marinade and the fish, neither overpowering the other.

Ingredients

- 3 pounds salmon fillets
- garlic powder, to taste
- lemon pepper, as per taste
- salt, as per taste
- 2/3 cup brown sugar
- 2/3 cup soy sauce
- 2/3 cup water
- 1/2 cup oil

Method

1. Sprinkle the garlic powder, lemon pepper and salt on the salmon fillets.

2. Combine the brown sugar, vegetable oil, soy sauce and water in a small bowl. Keep stirring until the sugar melts. Place the seasoned salmon filets in a large re-sealable bag and pour the prepared marinade mix onto it. Shake the bag to coat and refrigerate for 2 hours.

3. Turn the grill up to medium heat and let it preheat. Spray the cooking spray on the grill. Place the marinated salmon on the grill and cook for 8 minutes per side or until the fish flakes away when cut with a fork. Serve hot!

Tips/Notes

Salmon is considered to be one of the healthiest fishes in the world as it is extremely rich in vitamin B12, amino acids, proteins and omega-3 fatty acids. Serve it with a side of a salad and you've got a highly nutritional meal on your hands.

128. Delicious Black Bean Patties

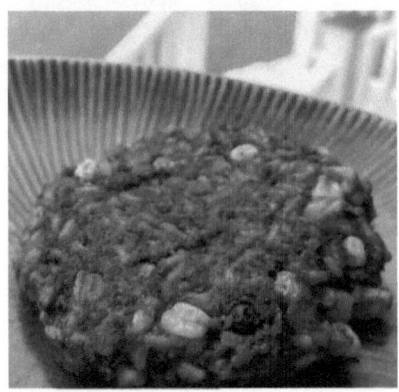

Take a break from the frozen veggie burgers and try this recipe; you will never go back to the frozen aisle for these again!

Ingredients

- 1 onion, finely chopped
- 2 (16 ounce) cans black beans, drained and rinsed
- 2 tablespoons chili powder
- 2 teaspoons Thai chili sauce or hot sauce
- 1 green bell pepper, finely chopped
- 6 cloves garlic, finely chopped
- 1 cup bread crumbs
- 2 eggs
- 2 tablespoons cumin

Method

1. Turn up your grill to high heat and spray some cooking spray on the grill. Place a piece of aluminum foil on it. Add the black beans to a medium sized bowl and mash them using a fork until they are thick and mushy. Add the onion, bell pepper and garlic to it and mix well.

2. Combine the egg, cumin, chili powder and chili sauce together in a small bowl. Pour this mix into the black bean mix and mix well. Add in the bread crumbs and mix until the mixture can hold together.

3. Divide the mix into 8 patties. Place the patties on the foil and grill for about 8 minutes on each side. Place in burger buns and serve immediately or refrigerate for later use.

Tips/Notes

Black beans aid the digestive system and reduces the risk of colon cancer! Also, soaking the black beans overnight helps increase their advantageous properties' just make sure you use the soaking water in your cooking too; after all, even the water is rich in leached nutrients.

129. Honey Chicken and Vegetable Skewers

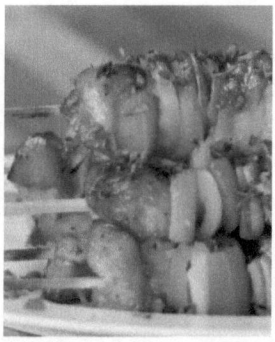

This sweet and tangy recipe is loved by all! You can substitute the usual components of an outdoor barbeque with this delicious and fresh recipe.

Ingredients

- 2 tablespoons vegetable oil
- 8 teaspoons honey
- 8 teaspoons soy sauce
- 1/8 teaspoon ground black pepper
- 4 chicken breast halves, skinless and boneless - cut into 1-inch cubes
- 1 clove garlic
- 1 medium onion, cut into cubes
- 2 small red bell pepper, cut into cubes
- Skewers

Method

1. Combine the honey, black pepper, soy sauce and vegetable oil together in a large bowl. Spoon out a few teaspoons of the marinade into a smaller bowl and add the chicken pieces to the big bowl. Add in the red bell peppers, garlic and onion to the chicken and mix well. Refrigerate the bowl overnight or for at least 2 hours.

2. Turn the grill up on high heat and preheat. Drain the excess marinade and discard it. Skewer the chicken pieces and vegetables on the skewers, alternately.

3. Spray the grill with some cooking spray and place the skewers on the grill. Cook the skewers for about 150 minutes, constantly turning and brushing with the marinade set aside. Serve hot!

Tips/Notes

According to researchers, the cooking of meats over an open flame has had a catalytic effect on the evolution of the human brain! Keep barbequing!

130. Chicken Tikka Masala

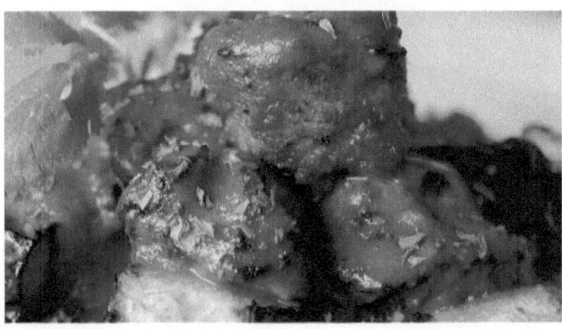

Chicken Tikka Masala is a chicken steeped in a blend of spices and yogurt and served in a tomato based cream sauce. This dish is best served with a side of pita bread or on a bed of steamed rice.

Ingredients

- 2 cups yogurt
- 2 tablespoons lemon juice
- 4 teaspoons ground cumin
- 2 teaspoons ground cinnamon

- 4 teaspoons cayenne pepper
- 4 teaspoons black pepper, freshly ground
- 2 tablespoons fresh ginger, minced
- 8 teaspoons salt, or to taste
- 6 chicken breasts, skinless and boneless, cut into bite-size pieces
- 8 long skewers
- 2 tablespoons butter
- 2 cloves garlic, minced
- 2 jalapeno peppers, finely chopped
- 4 teaspoons ground cumin
- 4 teaspoons paprika
- 2 tablespoons salt, or to taste
- 2 cups canned tomato sauce
- 2 cups heavy cream
- 1/2 cup chopped fresh cilantro

Method

1. Mix together the lemon juice, yogurt, cinnamon, cumin, black pepper, cayenne pepper, salt and ginger in a large bowl. Add in the chicken and cover with cling wrap. Refrigerate for an hour.

2. Turn up your grill on high and preheat. Spray the grill with some cooking spray. Skewer the chicken pieces on the skewers and discard the excess marinade. Place on the grill and cook for 7 minutes on each side.

3. In a large skillet, melt the butter over a medium flame. Add the garlic and jalapeno and sauté for 1 minute. Add in the paprika, cumin and salt. Pour in the tomato sauce and heavy cream and mix well. Once the gravy starts simmering, lower the heat and cook until the sauce thickens. Add in the grilled pieces of chicken and cook for another 10 minutes. Serve hot topped with some cilantro!

Tips/Notes

The grilled pieces of chicken are known as "tikkas" and are traditionally baked in a clay oven known as a tandoor.

131. Tangy Grilled Chicken

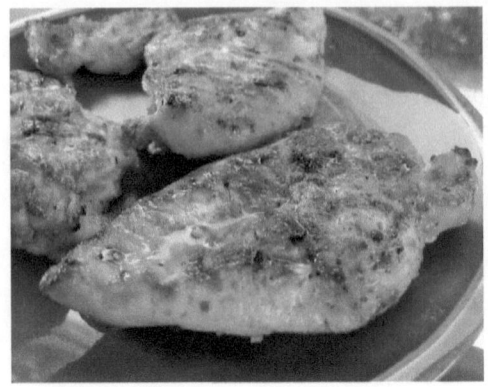

This easy to make dish is sweet and tangy and will end up as your and your family's favorite dish!

Ingredients

- 8 chicken breast halves, skinless and boneless
- 2 teaspoons steak sauce
- 2/3 cup Dijon mustard
- 1/4 cup mayonnaise
- 1/2 cup honey

Method

1. Turn up the grill on medium heat and let it preheat. Spray with some cooking oil.

2. Combine the steak sauce, mustard, mayonnaise and honey in a bowl. Spoon out some for basting and add the chicken to the remaining marinade. Coat well and allow marinating for 30 minutes.

3. Set up the grill to indirectly heat and cook the chicken for about 20 minutes, turning the chicken on occasion. With each turn baste the chicken with the reserved marinade. Serve immediately!

Tips/Notes

Mayonnaise is a base for a variety of other sauces. For example, tartar sauce is a combination of pickled onions, mayonnaise and cucumber. Ranch dressing is prepared by combining buttermilk, finely minced onion and mayonnaise together.

132. Stuffed Jalapenos Wrapped in Bacon

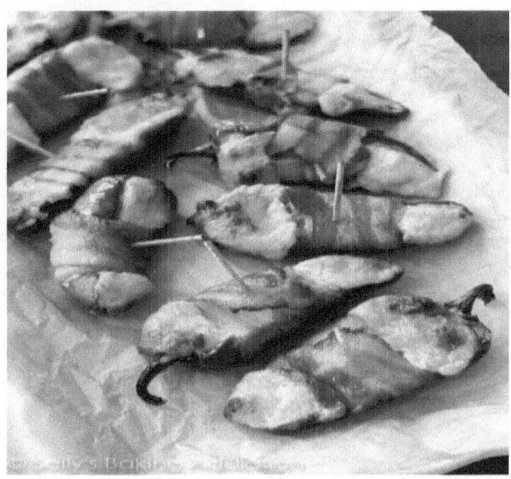

Cream cheese stuffed jalapenos, covered with bacon and grilled to perfection!

Ingredients

- 12 fresh jalapeno peppers, cut into halves and seeds removed
- 2 (8 ounce) packages cream cheese
- 24 slices bacon

Method

1. Turn the grill up to high heat and spray it with cooking spray.

2. Spoon the cream cheese into the jalapeno halves and wrap the bacon around the jalapeno halves. Keep in place using a toothpick.

3. Place the prepared jalapenos on the grill and grill until the bacon is crispy. Serve hot!

Tips/Notes

Jalapenos were the first peppers sent to space!

133. Grilled Garlic and Pepper Shrimp

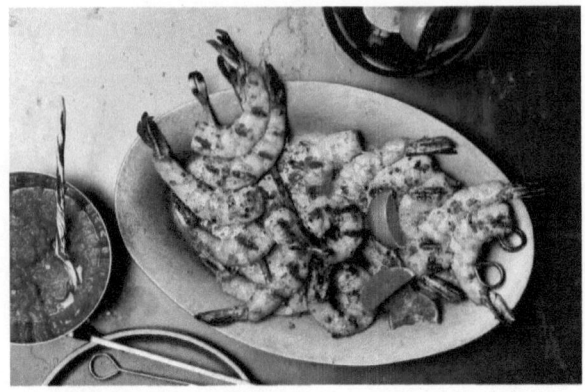

This delicious dish is best served on a bed of freshly prepared pasta!

Ingredients

- 2 lemons, juiced
- 2 cups extra virgin olive oil
- 2 tablespoons tomato paste
- 2 teaspoons ground black pepper
- 4 tablespoons hot pepper sauce
- 1/2 cup fresh parsley, chopped
- 2 teaspoons salt
- 6 cloves garlic, minced
- 4 teaspoons dried oregano
- 4 pounds large shrimp, peeled and deveined with tails attached
- Skewers

Method

1. Combine the lemon juice, olive oil, tomato paste, black pepper, hot pepper sauce, parsley, salt, garlic and oregano together in a bowl. Spoon out some of the marinade and reserve for basting. Pour the marinade into a large re-sealable bag and add in the shrimp. Seal and shake to coat. Refrigerate for 2 hours.

2. Turn up your grill to medium high and coat the grill with some cooking spray. Drain the shrimp and thread them onto the skewers.

3. Place the shrimp on the grill and cook for 7 minutes per side. Frequently baste using the reserved marinade. Cook until opaque and serve hot.

Tips/Notes

To easily peel garlic just pop them into the microwave for 5 – 10 seconds. The skin will pop off and the flesh will become softer, making it easier to crush or mince it!

134. Honey Garlic Steaks

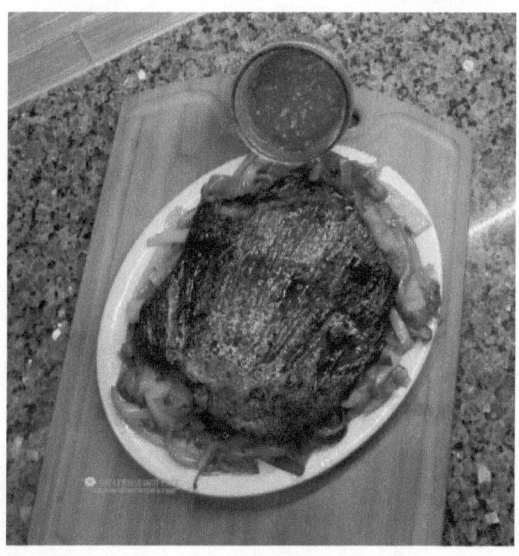

This delicious recipe gives you a delicious piece of savory steak that is so succulent it almost melts in the mouth!

Ingredients

- 1 cup balsamic vinegar
- 1/2 cup soy sauce
- 6 tablespoons minced garlic
- 4 tablespoons honey
- 4 tablespoons olive oil
- 4 teaspoons ground black pepper
- 2 teaspoons Worcestershire sauce
- 2 teaspoons onion powder
- 1 teaspoon salt
- 1 teaspoon liquid smoke flavoring
- 2 pinches cayenne pepper
- 4 (1/2 pound) rib-eye steaks

Method

1. Combine the soy sauce, vinegar, garlic, olive oil, honey, Worcestershire sauce, black pepper, salt, onion powder, cayenne pepper and liquid smoke in a bowl.

2. Place the steaks in the marinade and slowly rub the marinade into the steaks. Cover and refrigerate for 2 days. Turn up the grill to medium high and preheat. Spray cooking spray on the grill.

3. Place the steaks on the preheated grill and cook for about 7 minutes per side for a medium piece of steak. Serve hot with a side of grilled vegetables and mashed potatoes!

Tips/Notes

It is better to over season a steak while grilling as there is high probability that all the heavy seasoning will fall off the steak into the fire while you grill, resulting in an under seasoned steak.

135. Butter Basil Shrimp

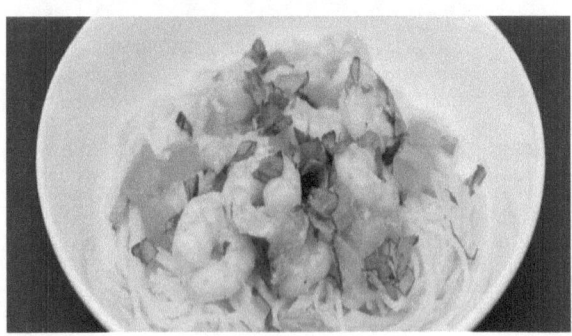

The buttery goodness, when combined with the strong flavors of mustard and basil create a tantalizing magic of flavors on your tongue!

Ingredients

- 4 teaspoons extra virgin olive oil
- 8 teaspoons butter, melted
- 1 lemon, juiced
- 5 teaspoons Dijon mustard
- 1/4 cup fresh basil leaves, minced
- 2 cloves garlic, minced

- salt to taste
- white pepper, to taste
- 2 pounds fresh shrimp, peeled and deveined
- Skewers

Method

1. Combine the melted butter, olive oil, mustard, lemon juice, garlic and basil in a shallow dish. Season to taste with white pepper and salt. Add in the shrimps and toss well until well coated. Cover the dish and refrigerate for an hour or two.

2. Turn up the grill to high and spray the grill with some cooking spray. Drain the shrimp and thread them onto the skewers. Discard the extra marinate.

3. Place the skewers on the grill and cook for about 5 minutes, frequently turning. Serve hot!

Tips/Notes

Basil is not only one of the healthiest herbs, with a rich content of vitamin A, but also is considered to be a holy plant in India, with women praying to it and watering it first thing every morning!

136. London Broil

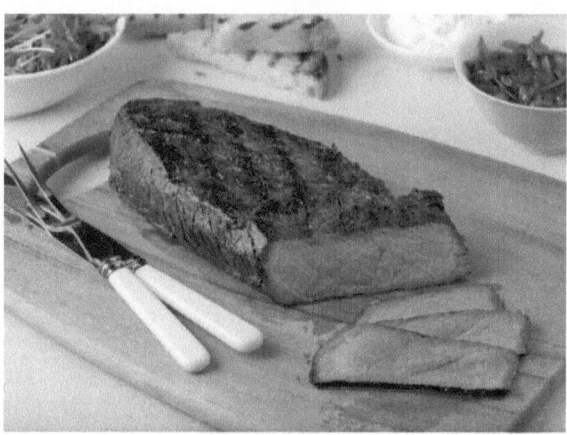

The steak is so juicy, succulent and flavorful on its own; you won't feel the need to accompany it with condiments of any kind!

Ingredients

- 1/2 clove garlic, minced
- 1/2 teaspoon salt
- 4 1/2 teaspoons soy sauce
- 1 1/2 teaspoons ketchup
- 1 1/2 teaspoons vegetable oil
- 1/4 teaspoon ground black pepper
- 1/4 teaspoon dried oregano
- 2 pounds flank steak

Method

1. Combine the salt, garlic, ketchup, soy sauce, black pepper, vegetable oil and oregano in a small bowl.

2. Rub the prepared marinate on the steak flanks and wrap in an aluminum foil. Refrigerate overnight, turning the steak over every few hours. Turn up the grill to high and lightly grease the grill.

3. Place the marinated steak on the grill and cook for about 7 minutes for a medium steak. Rest the steak for 5 minutes before slicing. Serve hot!

Tips/Notes

The London Broil originated in North America and is fairly unknown in the city it is named after!

137. Grilled Fish Tacos with A Zesty Lemon Dressing

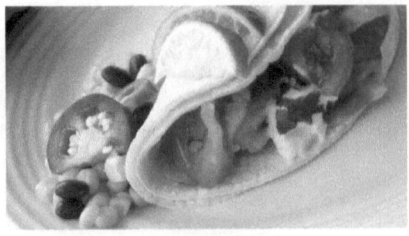

These grilled fish tacos make for an ideal meal and taste delicious when served accompanied with a chipotle lime dressing that not only enhances the flavor of the tacos, but also add some zing to them! You can add or remove the toppings as per your taste.

Ingredients

- 1/2 cup extra virgin olive oil
- 2 teaspoons seafood seasoning
- 1 tablespoon honey
- 1/4 cup distilled white vinegar
- 4 teaspoons lime zest
- 1/4 cup fresh lime juice
- 2 teaspoons hot pepper sauce, or to taste
- 4 cloves garlic, minced
- 1 teaspoon chili powder
- 1 teaspoon cumin
- 1 teaspoon ground black pepper
- 2 pounds tilapia fillets, cut into chunks

Dressing

- 2 cups light sour cream
- 1 cup adobo sauce
- 1/4 cup fresh lime juice
- 4 teaspoons lime zest
- 1/2 teaspoon cumin
- 1/2 teaspoon chili powder
- 1 teaspoon seafood seasoning
- Salt, to taste
- Pepper, to taste

Toppings

- 2 (10 ounce) packages tortillas
- 3 large ripe tomatoes, diced
- 2 bunches cilantro, chopped finely
- 1 large cabbage, cored and shredded
- 4 limes, cut in wedges

Method

1. Combine the extra virgin olive oil, lime juice, vinegar, honey, lime zest, cumin, garlic, seafood seasoning, chili powder, hot sauce and black pepper in a bowl. Whisk until the marinade is well blended. Place the fish filets in a flat dish with raised sides and pour the

prepared marinade over fillets. Cover the dish with some plastic wrap and place in a refrigerator for 8 to 10 hours.

2. To prepare the dressing, whisk together the adobo sauce and sour cream in a bowl until well blended. Add in the lime zest, lime juice, chili powder, cumin and seafood seasoning and mix well. Taste and add salt and pepper as per needed. Cover the bowl and place in the refrigerator to chill.

3. Turn up your grill on high heat and leave to preheat. Lightly spray the grill with some cooking spray and place it about 4 inches above the flame.

4. Drain the fish from the marinade and discard the extra marinade. Place the marinated fish on the grill and cook for about 9 minutes, flipping over around the 4 and half minute mark or cook until the fish fillet easily flakes with a fork.

5. To assemble the tacos, place the grilled fish in the center of the tortillas. Top the fish with some chopped cilantro, cabbage and cilantro. Spoon some of the prepared dressing over the toppings and roll the tortillas around the fish and toppings. Serve immediately with some lemon wedges on the side.

Tips/Notes

The word taco means "light lunch" in Mexican Spanish and 3rd October is celebrated as National Taco Day.

138. Butter Beer Chicken

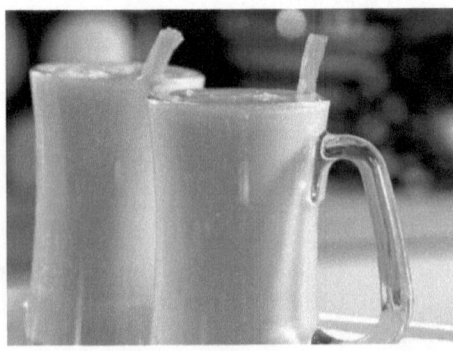

Cooking a whole chicken can often seem like a Herculean task, but the recipe makes the whole process as easy as snapping your fingers. The dish is a little unorthodox, but the final result is a delicious, moist and juicy meal! And despite the name, this chicken has nothing to do with the Harry Potter universe!

Ingredients

- 1/2 cup butter
- 6 ounces beer (discard the extra beer from the can)
- 1 tablespoon garlic salt
- 2-pound whole chicken
- 1 tablespoon paprika
- Salt, to taste
- Pepper, to taste

Method

1. Turn up your grill on a low heat and let the grill preheat. Heat a small skillet over a medium flame. Add in ¼ cup butter and melt it. Sprinkle in half the quantities of the garlic salt, salt, paprika and pepper in the melted butter and mix well.

2. Leave the beer in the can and pour in the remaining butter into the can with the beer. Add the remaining spices into the can. Once all the ingredients are in it, place the beer can on a use and throw baking sheet. Carefully place the chicken on the can by placing the can into the opening of the chicken. Using a pastry brush gently baste the chicken using the prepared seasoned melted butter mix.

3. Gently lift the baking sheet, ensuring that you do not disturb the placement of the can and the chicken, and place the baking sheet on the preheated grill. Cook the chicken on the low flame for about 3 to 3 and half hours or until a thermometer inserted in the center of the chicken reads 180 degrees Fahrenheit or about 80 degrees Celsius.

4. Just before serving, gently remove the can from the cavity. Take care; the can will be very hot, so use some sturdy tongs. Serve hot!

Tips/Notes

Beer contains a high level of silicone that helps in the strengthening of bones and contains almost all the nutrients that we need to survive.

139. Fiery Shrimp

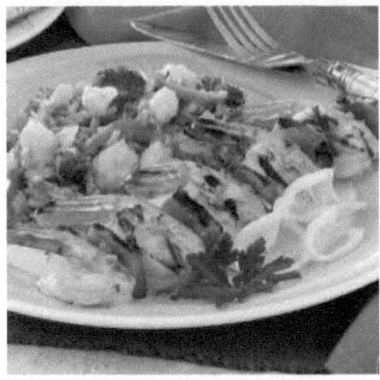

If you need a quick meal fix, these shrimps will make your ideal go to meal!

Ingredients

- 2 large cloves garlic
- 1 teaspoon cayenne pepper
- 4 pounds large shrimp, peeled and deveined
- 2 tablespoons coarse salt
- 1/4 cup olive oil
- 2 teaspoons paprika
- 4 teaspoons lemon juice
- 16 wedges lemon, for garnish

Method

1. Turn up your grill to medium heat to preheat. Place the garlic with the salt in a bowl and crush. Add in the cayenne, paprika, lemon juice and olive oil to make a paste. Place the shrimp in a large bowl, add in the spicy paste and toss to coat.

2. Grease the grate with some oil and place the shrimp on it. Cook for about 3 minutes per side or until the shrimp turn opaque. Serve hot, garnished with some lemon wedges.

Tips/Notes

Cayenne pepper aids in weight loss by reducing appetite, increasing energy usage in the body and also helps in breaking down the fats in the body!

140. Bacon Wrapped Hamburgers

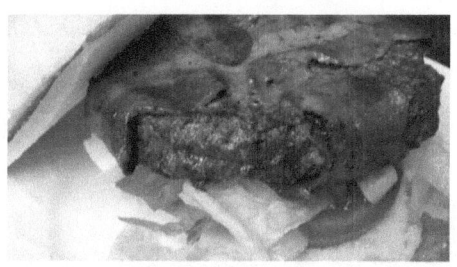

The name might sound weird, but the bacon in the patty makes the patty moist and tender!

Ingredients

- 1 cup Cheddar cheese, shredded
- 2 tablespoons Parmesan cheese, grated
- 2 small onions, finely chopped
- 2 eggs
- 2 tablespoons ketchup
- 2 tablespoons Worcestershire sauce
- 1 teaspoon salt
- 1/4 teaspoon pepper
- 2 pounds ground beef
- 12 slices bacon
- 12 hamburger buns, split

Method

1. Turn up your grill on high heat and let it preheat. Combine the Cheddar, Parmesan, eggs, onions, Worcestershire sauce, ketchup, pepper and salt in a large bowl, whisking well. Add in the ground beef, crumbling it into bits with your hands and mix well.

2. Divide into 12 equal parts and shape into patties. Take a slice of bacon and wrap it around the patty carefully, ensuring that you don't mess the shape of the patty. Fasten the bacon in place using a toothpick.

3. Grease the grill with some cooking spray and place the patties on it. Cook for about 7 minutes per side or until the beef is well cooked. Carefully remove the toothpick, place the patties in the buns and serve immediately.

Tips/Notes

Bacon contains a large amount of Choline, a compound that aids in the brain development in fetuses and 3rd September is International Bacon Day.

141. Grilled Zesty Tilapia with A Sweet and Spicy Mango Salsa

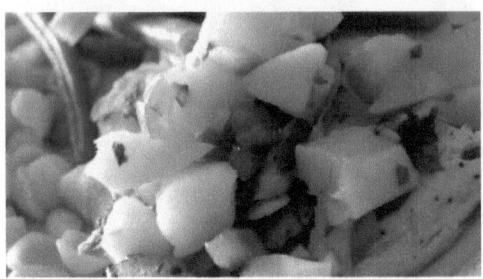

Do not let the exhaustive list of ingredients intimidate you, this dish is extremely easy to prepare! If you do not like mangoes or cannot find them in your local market, you can substitute the mango for strawberries!

Ingredients

- 2/3 cup extra virgin olive oil
- 2 tablespoons lemon juice
- 2 tablespoons fresh parsley, minced
- 2 cloves garlic, minced
- 2 teaspoons dried basil
- 2 teaspoons ground black pepper
- 1 teaspoon salt
- 4 (6 ounce) tilapia fillets

For the Mango Salsa

- 2 large ripe mangos, peeled, pit removed and diced
- 1 red bell pepper, diced
- 1/4 cup red onion, minced
- 2 tablespoons fresh cilantro, chopped
- 2 jalapeno peppers, seeded and minced
- 1/4 cup lime juice
- 2 tablespoons lemon juice
- Salt, to taste
- Pepper, to taste

Method

1. Combine the lemon juice, extra virgin olive oil, basil, garlic, salt and pepper in a bowl. Pour the prepared marinade in a re-sealable bag and add the tilapia fillets to the bag. Remove the excess air from the bag and seal it shut. Shake the bag up to coat the fillets with the marinade. Place the bag in the refrigerator for about 2 hours.

2. To prepare the mango salsa, place the chopped mango, red onion, red bell pepper, jalapeno peppers, and cilantro in a small bowl. Pour in the lemon juice and lime juice and mix well. Taste and season accordingly with salt and pepper. Pop into the refrigerator to chill. Turn up your grill to medium high heat and let it preheat for a few minutes. Lightly spray the grate with some cooking spray. Carefully remove the tilapia fillets from the marinade and lightly dab with an absorbent towel to get rid of the excess marinade.

3. Place the fillets on the preheated and prepared grill and grill for about 4 minutes per side or until the fish gets opaque in the center and easily flakes when flaked with a fork. To serve, place the grilled tilapia on a plate and spoon a healthy helping of the prepared mango salsa on the fillet. Serve immediately.

Tips/Notes

The mango is known as the "king of fruits" and is a rich source of vitamin A, vitamin B6, Vitamin C, vitamin E and copper.

142. Orange and Garlic Grilled Tuna

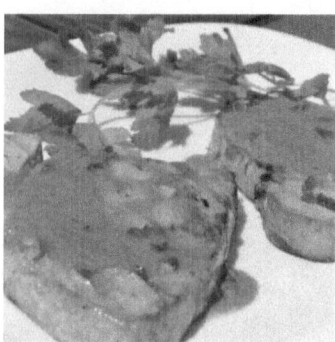

The tangy and savory combination of orange juice and garlic gives this dish a delicious and strong flavor.

Ingredients

- 1/2 cup orange juice
- 1/4 cup fresh parsley, chopped
- 1/2 cup soy sauce
- 2 tablespoons lemon juice
- 1/4 cup olive oil
- 1 teaspoon fresh oregano, chopped
- 2 cloves garlic, minced
- 1 teaspoon ground black pepper
- 8 (4 ounce) tuna steaks

Method

1. Combine the orange juice, olive oil, soy sauce, garlic, lemon juice, parsley, pepper and oregano in a large glass dish. Put the tuna steaks in the prepared marinade and flip over and over to coat well. Place the dish with the marinade and steaks in the refrigerator for about 30 minutes.

2. Turn up the grill to high heat and preheat. Lightly grease the grate with some oil. Place the marinated tuna steaks on the grill and keep the extra marinade. Cook the steak for about 5 minutes on one side, flip over, baste with the marinade and keep cooking until done. Serve hot!

Tips/Notes

Tuna is rich in protein, omega 3 fatty acids, vitamin D and Selenium. Selenium is a rarely found nutrient that plays an important role in boosting the immune system of the body.

143. Pineapple Chicken Tenders

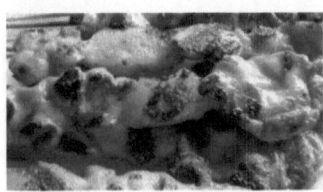

This recipe is ideal for the days when you want to have a light meal without heavy meats weighing you down.

Ingredients

- 4 pounds chicken breast or strips, cut into bite sized pieces
- 2 cups pineapple juice
- 2/3 cup light soy sauce
- 1 cup packed brown sugar
- Skewers

Method

1. Soak the skewers in some warm water for about 20 minutes. Drain and dry on an absorbent towel. Heat a small saucepan over a medium flame. Pour in the pineapple juice and let it heat through for a minute. Add in the soy sauce and brown sugar and mix well. Take the mixture of heat just before it starts boiling.

2. Put the chicken pieces in a medium sized bowl. Pour the pineapple mix over the chicken, completely covering the chicken. Cover the bowl using a plastic wrap and refrigerate for about 30 minutes, or more if possible. Turn up your grill to medium low heat and grease the grate with some oil or cooking spray. Skewer the marinated chicken pieces on the prepared skewers.

3. Place the chicken skewers on the prepared and preheated grill and cook for about 7 minutes per side or until the chicken is done. Watch the skewers closely, as the pineapple juice caramelizes quickly, resulting in easy burning. Serve hot!

Tips/Notes

Soy sauce is considered to be one of the oldest condiments of the world, and has been used to prepare dishes in China since almost 2,500 years now.

144. Pork Teriyaki Don

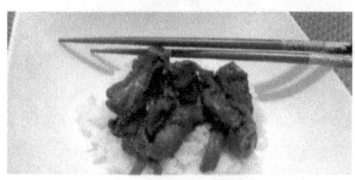

Pork tenderloins are good cuts of meat that you can use for this dish. Not only that it's lean and tender but it also cooks really fast.

Ingredients

- ½ cup of soy sauce
- ½ cup of mirin
- 3 tablespoons of sugar
- ½ teaspoon of ginger (grated)
- 350 grams of pork (tenderloins; cut to strips)
- 2 tablespoons of oil
- ¼ teaspoon of sesame oil
- 1 bell pepper (diced, can use green or red)
- Cooked rice for serving

Method

1. Combine soy sauce, sugar, mirin and ginger in a bowl. Add pork strips and toss it to evenly coat. Cover and cool in refrigerator for about 20 minutes.

2. Heat oil over medium to high heat inside a wok. Stir fry marinated pork for 1 minute then transfer on a plate. Set aside.

3. Pour on sesame oil and sauté the bell peppers. Put back the pork with the marinade and cook until done. Season to taste. Serve on top of cooked rice. Enjoy!

Tips/Notes

You can marinate your pork a night before cooking. That way flavors are more absorbed and infused on the meat itself.

145. Healthy Beef Broccoli Stir Fry

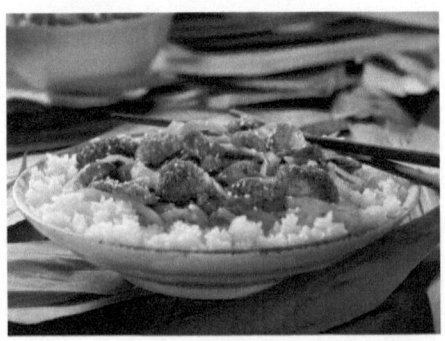

Tender, melt in your mouth beefy goodness paired with vibrant and crunchy broccoli is a surefire hit for your friends and family. Quick, easy and healthy – an all-time dish in a jiffy.

Ingredients

For the beef

- 300 grams of beef sirloin (sliced to 2x1 inches)
- ½ teaspoon of meat tenderizer
- 1 tablespoon of soy sauce
- 2 tablespoons of ginger juice
- ¼ teaspoon of salt
- A pinch of pepper
- 1 tablespoon of egg white
- 1 tablespoon of cornstarch
- 1 cup of cooking oil

For the broccoli

- 1 medium sized broccoli
- 1 tablespoon of oil
- 1 teaspoon of garlic

For stir frying

- 2 tablespoons of oil
- 1 piece of small ginger (pounded)
- 1 tablespoon of garlic (chopped)
- 1 stalk of leek (sliced to an inch-thick rings)
- 5 slices of carrots
- 12 pieces of snow peas
- 2 tablespoons of oyster sauce
- 2 tablespoons of gin
- ½ cup of chicken stock
- 1 tablespoon of cornstarch (dissolve it on 2 tablespoons of water)
- 1 tablespoon of sesame oil
- Salt, sugar and pepper for tasting

Method

1. To prepare the beef: mix beef and the meat tenderizer and let rest for about 5 minutes. Add soy sauce, salt, ginger juice and pepper.

Marinate it the whole night. Once you are ready to prepare the dish, mix the cornstarch and egg white to the meat. Heat oil inside the wok and start frying the beef for approximately 3 minutes. Set aside.

2. To prepare the broccoli: blanch it over boiling water until color changes. Place in a bowl of ice water to maintain crunchiness of veggie. Heat oil in a pan and sauté the garlic until fragrant. Add broccoli and mix them well. Transfer to a plate and set them aside.

3. Heat oil in the wok. Sauté ginger and garlic until it becomes fragrant. Mix in all other veggies, gin, oyster sauce and stock. Once it boils, add beef and continue to cook. Season to taste using sugar, pepper and salt. Use the cornstarch mixture to thicken the sauce. Once done add sesame oil. Pour the cooked mixture on top of the broccoli and serve. Enjoy!

Tips/Notes

To make the ginger juice, peel a small sized ginger and grate. Squeeze the grated ginger to get the juice and strain. This would make 2 tablespoons of ginger juice.

146. Tenderloin Strips with Lemongrass

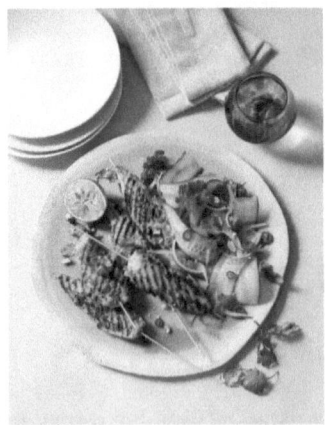

Are you in a hurry? Then stir frying is the best way to cook quick and healthy meals. Try this low-fat and protein packed recipe that is perfect for people in a hurry. Infused with cilantro and lemongrass, you will definitely enjoy the hint of Thai flavor.

Ingredients

- 1 ½ tablespoons of brown sugar
- 1 tablespoon of KecapManis (sweet soy sauce)
- 1 tablespoon of fish sauce
- ½ teaspoon of salt
- ¼ teaspoon of pepper
- 400 grams of beef tenderloin (sliced to 2 ½ inch thick strips)
- 1 tablespoon of cornstarch
- 2 tablespoons of cooking oil
- 1 medium sized red onions (thinly sliced)
- 2 teaspoons of garlic (chopped finely)
- 5 stalks of lemongrass (minced and trimmed)
- 1-2 pieces of bird's eye chili (chopped)
- 3 tablespoons of cilantro (chopped)
- Steamed rice for serving

Method

1. In a medium sized bowl, mix together kecapmanis, sugar, fish sauce, pepper and salt. Add the tenderloin strips and mix them well. Sprinkle it with cornstarch and combine them well. Marinate for about 15 minutes or if possible, do it overnight.

2. Heat the oil in a large sized wok over medium to high heat then sauté onions until cooked. Add the lemongrass and garlic and continue sautéing until they are fragrant. Add the beef with the marinade. Stir fry around 5-6 minutes or until beef is done depending on your preference. Add the chilies and stir continuously for a few seconds. Remove from heat and add the chopped cilantro. Mix it well. Serve immediately with the steamed rice and top it with cilantro leaves as garnish. Enjoy!

Tips/Notes

KecapManis is a sweet soy sauce used mostly in Indonesia and other Asian countries. It is thick, not salty and have rich caramel flavor. They are available on groceries and supermarkets.

147. Beef Stir Fry with Long Beans & Aromatic Paste

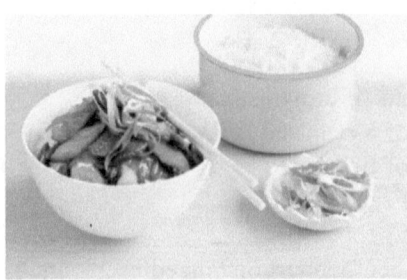

Now let me take you to the flavors of Thailand. A sumptuous and fragrant dish, this would liven up your palate and let you discover new and bold flavors.

Ingredients

- 2 tablespoons of oyster sauce
- 2 tablespoons of sugar (dark brown or you can use muscovado sugar if available)
- 1 tablespoon of fish sauce
- 350 grams of beef tenderloin (sliced to thin strips)

To prepare aromatic paste

- 1 stalk of lemongrass (minced and trimmed)
- 3 tablespoons of shallot (minced)
- 2 tablespoons of garlic (minced)
- 1 tablespoon of cilantro (minced)
- 2 teaspoons of Thai shrimp paste
- 1 teaspoon of ginger
- ½ teaspoon of chili flakes (optional)
- 5 pieces of black peppercorns
- 1 teaspoon of salt
- 3 tablespoons of vegetable oil
- 150 grams of string beans (cut into 1½ inch long, blanced)
- Pepper and salt for tasting
- 1-2 pieces of leaves of Kaffir lime (leaves thinly sliced; ribs discarded)
- Steamed rice (optional)

Method

1. In a medium sized bowl, make the marinade. Combine sugar, oyster sauce and fish sauce. Mix well until sugar is fully dissolved. Add the

beef and marinate for about 3-6 hours. But it's still best to marinate it overnight.

2. To make the aromatic paste, mix all of the ingredients in a large sized pestle and mortar. Pound the ingredients until achieving a smooth paste texture.

3. In a medium sized wok, heat the oil then sauté the aromatic paste for about a minute until fragrant. Add beef and its marinade and cook over medium high heat until the beef is cooked well and browned.

4. Add the blanched string beans and stir well. Season to taste then add the leaves of Kaffir lime. Remove from heat. Serve with rice if you want. Enjoy!

Tips/Notes

String beans are also called yard beans. They are a good source of folates and also have a good amount of Vitamin C that is good for the body.

148. Stir-fried Veggie Egg Noodles with Pork

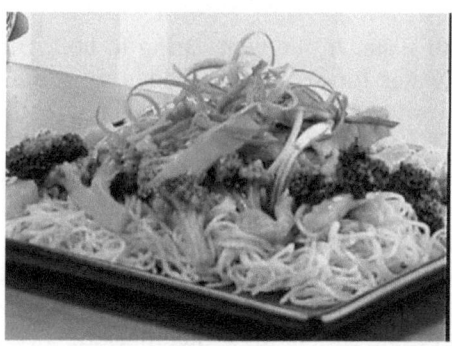

This is an appetizing noodle dish that would surely be a hit when you have visitors at home. It's quick and easy to prepare, easy on the budget and healthy for the body.

Ingredients

- 200 grams of egg noodles
- 1 tablespoon of canola oil
- 2 cloves of garlic (finely chopped)
- 100 grams of pork belly (sliced thinly and no skins)

- ½ cup leeks (thinly sliced, white part only)
- 2 tablespoons of cooking wine (Chinese variety)
- 1 cup of straw mushrooms (canned, drained and cut to half)
- 2 tablespoons of green onions (chopped)
- 2 tablespoons of cilantro

For the sauce

- 1 ½ tablespoons of oyster sauce

- 2 teaspoons of soy sauce

- 1 teaspoon of sugar

- 1 teaspoon of sesame oil

- Pepper and salt for tasting

- ½ cup of chicken stock or water if not available

Method

1. Put 4 cups of water in the wok. Bring to boil. Blanch the noodles in the boiling water for about 30 seconds to a minute then drain. Run through cold water and shake excess water.

2. To make the sauce: mix all the ingredients until sugar is well dissolved. Using same wok, heat oil over medium to high heat. Sauté garlic and add the pork belly. Stir fry until it turned light brown. Add cooking wine and leeks, stir well. Remove and set aside.

3. Pour the sauce and simmer over medium-high heat. Add pork mixture, mushrooms and noodles. Toss continuously to prevent from sticking on the wok. Stir well to coat the noodles evenly. Turn the heat off and add cilantro and green onions. Serve hot and enjoy!

Tips/Notes

You can substitute pork with chicken for a much healthier meat choice and lower calorie meal.

149. Stir-fried Vegetables Chinese Style

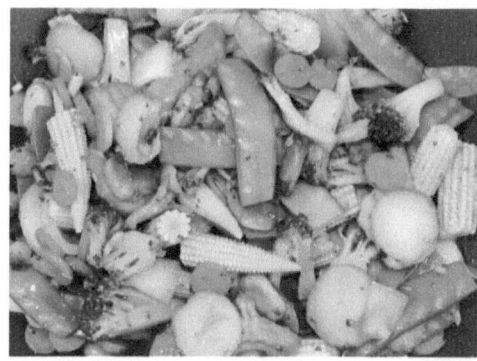

A delicious and colorful dish filled with healthy vegetables that are easy to cook in a jiffy.

Ingredients

- 2 tablespoons of vegetable oil
- ½ cup of red onion (sliced thinly)
- 200 grams of skinless pork belly (thinly sliced to an inch per piece
- 1 small sized zucchini (sliced into round sizes)
- 1 cup of cauliflower
- 1 medium sized carrots (sliced into round sizes)
- 1 eggplant (cut to an inch)
- 1 cup bell pepper (sliced)
- 1 clove garlic (minced)
- 1 teaspoon ginger (minced)
- ½ cup of oyster sauce
- 1 tablespoon of sugar (dissolve it in 2 tablespoons of water)
- 1 cup of green beans (trimmed)
- ¼ teaspoon of black pepper (ground)
- ¼ teaspoon of salt
- 2 tablespoons of sesame oil

Method

1. In a large size wok, heat oil over medium to high heat. Add the onions and stir continuously then add the pork until browned.

2. Add in the zucchini, carrots, cauliflower, bell pepper, eggplant, ginger, garlic and oyster sauce. Pour the sugar mixture and stir continuously. Cook for about 2 minutes.

3. Add the beans, salt and pepper for tasting. Cook well. Once done turn off heat then pour some sesame oil. Serve hot and enjoy!

Tips/Notes

Make sure to prep all your veggies ahead before cooking so can you can cook it quicker and faster.

150. Stir Fried Vermicelli with Chicken Teriyaki

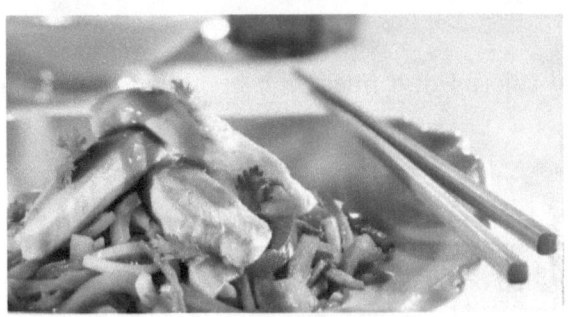

This is a complete meal that you would surely go back for more. Packed with proteins, carbohydrates and energy boosting ingredients, this would definitely satisfy any health-conscious individual.

Ingredients

- 500 grams of chicken fillet (breast part; cut into strips)

For the Teriyaki sauce

- 8 tablespoons of soy sauce (Japanese style)
- 2 tablespoons of sake (rice wine)
- 4 tablespoons of water
- 1 tablespoon of brown sugar
- 4 tablespoons of white sugar
- 1 ½ teaspoon of garlic (chopped finely)
- 1 1/2 teaspoon of ginger (grated)

For the vermicelli noodles

- 200 grams of vermicelli noodles
- 1 liter of boiling water
- 1 tablespoon of sesame oil

- 250 grams of snow peas (remove strings)
- 200 grams of red cabbage (shredded)
- 1 teaspoon of garlic (chopped finely)
- 1 tablespoon of hoisin sauce
- 1 tablespoon of soy sauce (light variety)
- 2 tablespoons of water
- Ground black pepper
- Sesame seeds (if desired)

Method

1. Prepare the teriyaki sauce by combining all the ingredients. Make sure to mix them all well. Once done, place the chicken strips and marinate for 1-3 hours.

2. Start cooking vermicelli noodles by putting them on a heat-resistant bowl and adding boiling water. Soak and cover noodles for about 3-5 minutes. Using the fork, separate noodles, drain and set aside.

3. To cook chicken, heat the grill to high. Spread a few oil and grill chicken for about 5 minutes. Brush the chicken with the marinade on both sides while cooking. Once done, put them on a plate and set aside.

4. In a large sized wok, heat oil over medium to high heat. Add garlic with the red cabbage and stir fry for about 2 minutes. Add hoisin sauce, water, soy sauce and cook for about 1-2 minutes.

5. Put snow peas and simmer until it becomes crisp and light green. Add noodles and toss to evenly spread the flavors. Once done transfer to plate. Place the grilled chicken on top of the noodles. If desired, sprinkle some sesame seeds. Serve hot and enjoy!

Tips/Notes

Vermicelli noodles are thin forms of rice noodles. They are used commonly as stir fried for Pad Thai, toppings on salads or soups like Vietnamese Pho. They are cholesterol free, fat free and has low sodium content.

151. Shrimp Chili Stir Fry

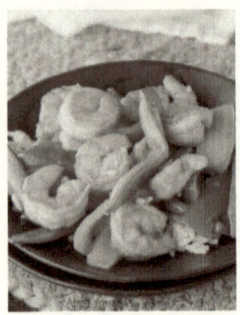

If you are a fan of food with a bit of heat, try this fast and delicious shrimp recipe to liven up the palates. Best with wine or a few beers with some friends on a Super Bowl or Boxing night.

Ingredients

- 300 grams of shrimp (deveined and shelled)
- 1 tablespoon of soy sauce (light variety)
- 2 tablespoons of oil
- 1 tablespoon of onion (chopped)
- 1 tablespoon of garlic (chopped)
- 2 pieces of bird's eye chili (chopped)
- 1/3 cup of bell pepper, red (cubed)
- 1/3 cup of bell pepper, green (cubed)
- 1/3 cup of bell pepper, yellow (cubed)
- 1 stalk of leeks (shredded)

To prepare the sauce

- 1 tablespoon of chili-garlic sauce
- 1 tablespoon of oyster sauce
- 1 tablespoon of gin
- ½ cup of chicken stock
- 1 tablespoon of water
- 1 tablespoon of cornstarch dissolved in 2 teaspoons of water
- 1 tablespoon of sesame oil

Method

1. Marinate the shrimp in salt, soy sauce and pepper. Put inside the refrigerator. To prep the sauce, combine all the ingredients and mix well. Set aside.

2. In a wok, stir fry the onions, chili and garlic. Add shrimps and the bell peppers. When the shrimp starts curling and turning orange, pour the sauce. Season with pepper, sugar and salt. Thicken it with the cornstarch mixture and add some sesame oil. Remove from heat. Serve with shredded leeks on top. Enjoy!

Tips/Notes

It's always best to buy the shrimps on the day you will be cooking them because the fresher the ingredients, the better!

152. Chicken Rice Indian Style

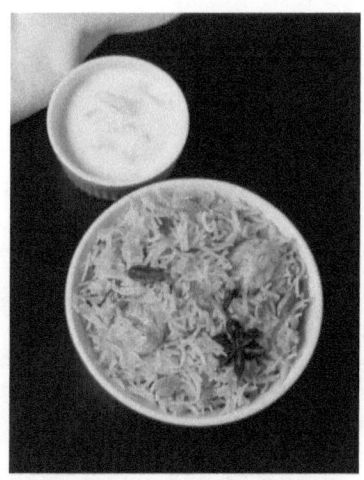

Expand and try out these other fried rice varieties using exotic and fragrant Indian spices. You will surely love them!

Ingredients

- 2 tablespoons of butter (unsalted)
- 2 tablespoons of onion (chopped)
- 1 teaspoon of garlic (minced)
- 2 pieces of chicken breast (fillet part, cubed)
- ½ teaspoon of cumin (ground)
- 2 teaspoon of curry powder
- 1 teaspoon of turmeric (ground)
- ¼ cup of frozen peas
- ¼ cup of raisins
- 4 cups of brown rice (cooked; you can also use red rice)

- Pepper and salt for tasting
- 3 tablespoons of almonds (slivered and toasted)

Method

1. Heat the butter and sauté the garlic and onions. Add the chicken and cook thoroughly. Add curry powder, cumin and turmeric. Mix them well.

2. Add peas and raisins then combine it with the cooked rice and stir fry until well coated with the spices. Season to taste. Once done remove from heat. Put in serving bowls and top it with almonds. Serve hot and enjoy!

Tips/Notes

This rice bowl will go perfectly with other grilled meats or vegetables.

153. Quick Stir-Fried Water Spinach with Pork Rind

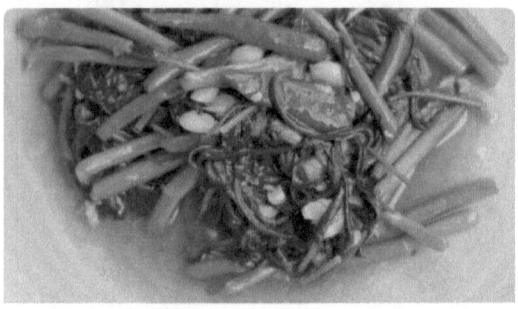

A tasty vegetable dish with a few indulgent pork cracklings for added crunch and exciting flavors.

Ingredients

- 5 teaspoons of oil
- 2 teaspoons of garlic (minced)
- 2 tablespoons of shrimp paste
- 300 grams of water spinach (separate leaves and stem)
- 4 teaspoons of vinegar
- 2 teaspoons of water
- 2 pieces of pork rind (crumbled)

Method

1. Heat the oil and sauté garlic in a medium sized wok or pan. Add shrimp paste and stir fry for a minute.

2. Add water spinach stems and cook until turned bright green in color. Add the leaves and cook it until it is wilted.

3. Pour the water and vinegar. Bring to boil and remove from fire. Transfer the veggies to a plate and top it with crumbled pork rind. Serve and enjoy.

Tips/Notes

Pork rinds are often called "chicharon" – a crispy pork crackling that are packed and can be readily bought in specialty supermarkets or Asian stores. If you can't find these pork rinds you can substitute it with any crispy chicken skins or bacon that you can make on your own.

154. Brown Rice with Stir-Fried Beef Teriyaki

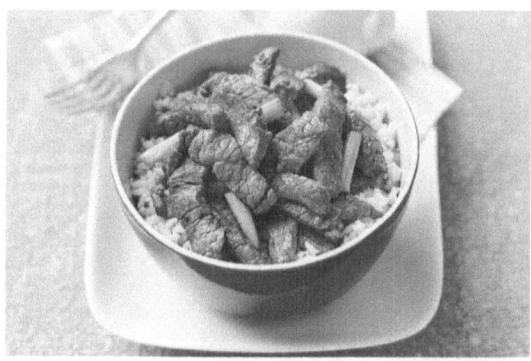

Here's another rice dish that you can check out. Healthy, quick and a good idea for people on the go.

Ingredients

- 2 teaspoons of cornstarch
- 3 tablespoons of teriyaki sauce
- 4 tablespoons of olive oil
- 500 grams of beef tenderloin (cut to thinly sliced strips)
- ½ cup of carrots (diced)
- ¼ cup green beans (blanched)

- 1 cup of baby corn (boiled)
- 3 cups of brown rice (cooked)

Method

1. Combine teriyaki sauce, cornstarch and 2 tablespoons of oil in a small sized bowl. Add beef and marinate it for about 45 minutes. Put it inside the refrigerator.

2. In a medium sized pan, stir fry green beans, baby corn and carrots with the remaining oil for about 2-3 minutes. Transfer on a plate.

3. Using the same pan, stir-fry the beef for about 3 minutes until it is tender. Bring back the vegetables and continue to stir fry for another 1-2 minutes. Remove from heat. Serve over the cooked rice and enjoy!

Tips/Notes

In this dish, you may also use the sukiyaki cut beef instead of the beef tenderloin.

155. Two Sauce Pork Tenders Stir Fry

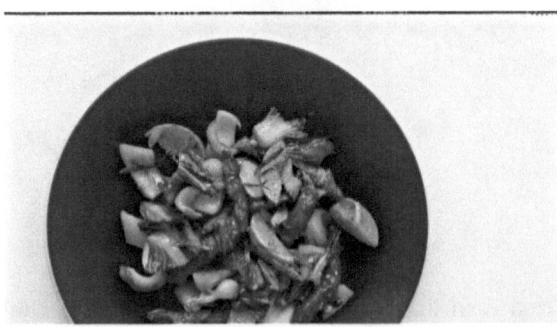

This is one dish that will gratify two tastes – one with a creamy mushroom sauce and the other spicy and sweet for a little kick on the palate!

Ingredients

For the pork tenders

- 1 ½ table spoons of oil
- 2 teaspoons of garlic powder

- 2 teaspoons of onion powder
- 1 ½ teaspoons of soy sauce
- 1 kilo of pork tenderloin (sliced to ¼ inch size)

To prepare sweet & spicy sauce

- 2 tablespoons of oil
- 1 tablespoon of garlic (minced)
- 1 onion (sliced)
- 1 red bell pepper (sliced)
- 1 green bell pepper (sliced)
- ½ cup of sweet chili sauce
- A dash of cayenne pepper

To prepare mushroom sauce

- ¼ cup of butter
- 1 teaspoon of garlic (minced)
- 1 small size canned mushrooms (sliced)
- 1 bottle of prepared gravy
- 1 teaspoon of Worcestershire sauce
- ½ teaspoon of soy sauce

Method

1. To prepare pork tenders: combine all the ingredients in a medium sized bowl and place the pork tenders on it. Marinate for about 15 minutes and divide it to 2 portions. Set aside.

2. To prepare the sweet & spicy sauce: heat oil in wok and sauté the onion and garlic. Add bell peppers and half of the marinated pork tenders. Stir fry until the pork is cooked thoroughly. Pour the sweet chili sauce and a dash of cayenne pepper and salt. You can adjust the heat depending on your taste.

3. To prepare the mushroom sauce: Melt butter on a different pan and sauté garlic. Add the rest of the pork tenders and cook well. Stir in gravy and mushrooms and bring to boil. Season with Worcestershire sauce and soy sauce. Simmer until cooked thoroughly. Prepare cooked rice in a bowl. Top it with preferred sauce and you are good to go. Enjoy!

Tips/Notes

The bottle of gravy in this recipe can be replaced using the canned cream of mushroom. Just use half of it and mix with a few cups of water and you will be able to prepare a creamy mushroom sauce.

156. Bell Pepper and Squid Stir Fry

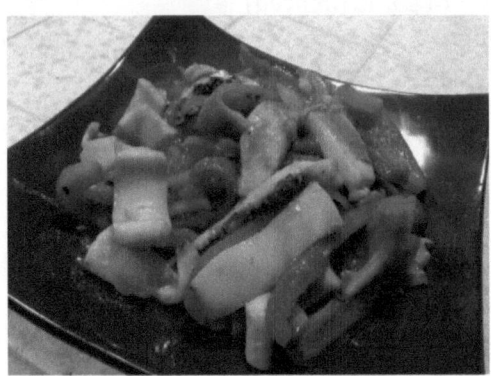

This easy squid stir fry can also be used as a perfect topping for your egg noodles or rice meal.

Ingredients

- 1 kilo of squid
- 1 tablespoon of hot bean paste
- 2 tablespoons of soy sauce
- 1 tablespoon of rice wine
- 2 teaspoons of sesame oil
- 1 teaspoon of salt
- 1 tablespoon of oil
- 2 tablespoons of garlic (minced)
- 1 teaspoon of garlic (minced)
- 1/3 cup of bell pepper, red (sliced to strips)
- 1/3 cup of bell pepper, green (sliced to strips)
- 1/3 cup of bell pepper, yellow (sliced to strips)
- Toasted sesame seeds

Method

1. Clean the squid, separate the heads from their bodies. Set aside and keep the squid heads. Peel the skin off their bodies and wash well.

Score each squid and make a crisscross pattern on the body. Cut for about 2x2 inch squares.

2. In a small saucepan, bring water to a boil. Drop the squid and let it boil once again. Quickly remove the squid and set aside. In a medium sized bowl, mix hot bean paste, rice wine, soy sauce, salt and sesame oil. Set aside.

3. Heat the wok and add oil. Sauté ginger and garlic. Add bell pepper strips and squid. Stir fry for about a minute then add the hot bean paste. Simmer for a few minutes. Serve hot and top it with cilantro and toasted sesame seeds. Enjoy!

Tips/Notes

When scoring, use a thin, sharp knife to make those cuts. Make sure that you don't cut through the squid meat.

157. Thai-style Prawn Salad

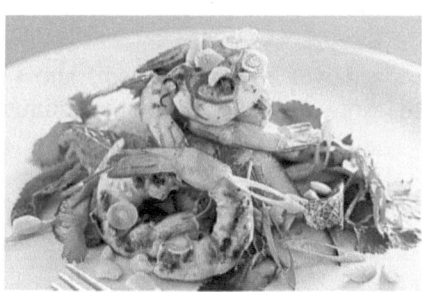

Another Asian inspired cuisine that captures the taste of Thailand. You can serve this dish either hot or cold – any which way, it's delicious!

Ingredients

- 200 grams of vermicelli noodles
- 1 tablespoon of oil
- 2 cloves of garlic (chopped)
- 1 piece of ginger (finely chopped)
- 1 piece of bird's eye chili (seeded, finely chopped)
- 450 grams of prawns (peeled, deveined, tails intact)
- 2 cups of snow peas
- 8 pieces of baby corn (halved in lengthwise)
- 4 stalks of spring onions (thinly sliced)

- 1 tablespoon of sesame seeds (toasted)
- 1 stalk of lemongrass (shredded thinly)

Dressing preparation

- 1 tablespoon of spring onions (chopped)
- 1 tablespoon of fish sauce
- 1 teaspoon of soy sauce
- 3 tablespoons of oil
- 1 teaspoon of sesame oil
- 2 tablespoons of rice vinegar

Method

1. Place the noodles in a large sized bowl. Pour boiling water over until fully immersed. Soak for about 5 minutes. Drain the noodles and refresh in cold water. Drain and set aside.

2. In a bottle or a bowl, mix all the ingredients for the dressing and combine them well.

3. In a medium sized wok or pan, heat oil and sauté garlic, chili and ginger. Add the prawns. Cook for about 3 minutes until it changes in color.

4. Stir in the snow peas, spring onions, sesame seed and baby corn. Toss it lightly and mix well.

5. Arrange the drained noodles in a serving plate. Top it with the cooked prawns. Drizzle with the prepared dressing. Serve and garnish with shredded lemon grass. Enjoy!

Tips/Notes

The quickest way in making vinaigrette is to put all ingredients in a bottle, tightly cover it and shake it well. By keeping it in a bottle, you can easily use it again for other salad dishes.

158. Fried Rice Oriental

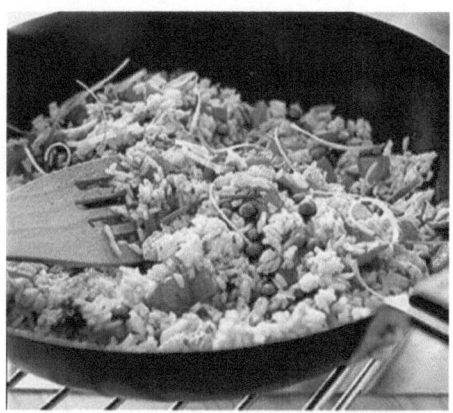

This fried rice is packed with veggies and meat that makes it a complete, satisfying meal by itself.

Ingredients

- 2 tablespoons of oil
- 1 tablespoon of garlic (chopped)
- 1 onion (chopped)
- 500 grams of ground chicken
- 2 pieces of chorizo (Chinese style, minced)
- 1 cup of mixed vegetables (frozen packed)
- 1 tablespoon of garlic chili sauce
- 3 tablespoons of soy sauce
- 4 tablespoons of hoisin sauce
- 6 cups of rice (cooked)
- Sugar, pepper and salt for tasting
- 1 teaspoon of sesame oil

Method

1. Heat the oil in a medium sized wok. Sauté onions and the garlic. Add chorizos and ground chicken. Stir fry until chicken is cooked.

2. Add in the vegetables. Season with the garlic chili sauce, hoisin and soy sauce.

3. Add cooked rice. Mix well until evenly coated. Season according to your preferred taste. Drizzle with the sesame season. Serve hot and enjoy!

Tips/Notes

You can make a seafood variation by substituting chicken and chorizo with shrimps, crabmeat and squid.

159. Pickled Eggs

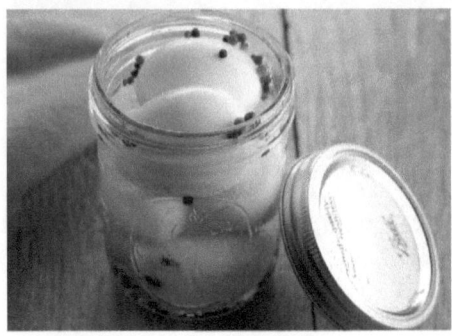

For the first recipe, we chose a very simple but very surprising recipe that most people have not even heard of. At least not in reference to pickles.

Ingredients

- 4 to 6 eggs
- Pickled beet juice

Method

1. Place the eggs in a saucepan of appropriate size, cover with water by 1 inch and bring it to simmer.

2. Cover the saucepan, remove it from the heat and allow to cool for 8 to 10 minutes. Drain the water, peel the eggs and place them in a jar.

3. Fill the jar with the beet juice, close it and put it in the refrigerator for up to one week

Tips/Notes

If it was really the taste the reason behind removing the eggs from your dietary habits, this is an interesting way to change your mind. If it suites your purposes further, you may experiment with the beet juice replacing it with vinaigrette as done in East Asia.

160. Tarragon Egg Salad

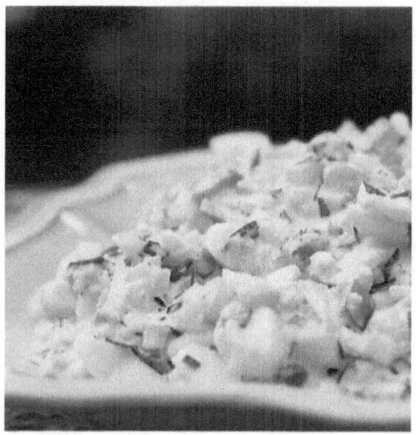

Many people prefer to include eggs in salads. The next couple of recipes will give you some more options than the usual ones. The following one is a most nutritious mix of 25 different micronutrients needed by the human body.

Ingredients

- 4 eggs
- 1 chopped shallot
- 1 teaspoon vinegar from white wine
- 3 tablespoons mayo
- Salt and pepper

Method

1. Hard cook the eggs the way you want them. Peel and chop to small pieces

2. Introduce into a bowl all the above ingredients and mix. Serve on pumpernickel bread.

Optional

An even more nutritious and satisfying salad can be enjoyed if the serving includes sliced cucumbers. This salad is a better option during the summer time.

161. Egg-mushroom Salad

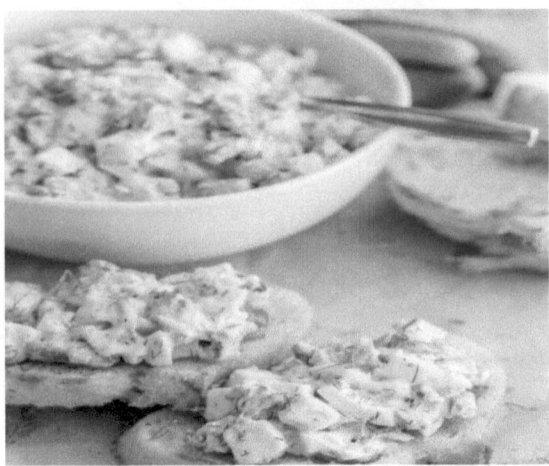

If the previous salad included 25 essential nutrients, this one will supply the human body with even more. And this is the point of the exercise. Nourish the body with what it actually needs. Not calories.

Ingredients

- 4 eggs
- 2 cups sliced mushrooms
- 1/3 cup olive oil
- 1 cup onion, chopped
- 2 tablespoons sour cream
- Salt, pepper and as much chopped parsley as you want

Method

1. Hard cook the eggs and chop them. Fry the mushrooms with the oil and the onion. Mix everything in a bowl and serve on rye toast.

Olive Oil

The reason that the Mediterranean diet has been characterized as arguably the most successful one, is the use of olive oil not only in its raw form, but also cooked. It's considered one of the superfoods containing a multitude of essential micronutrients including the monounsaturated fats.

162. Scalloped Eggs

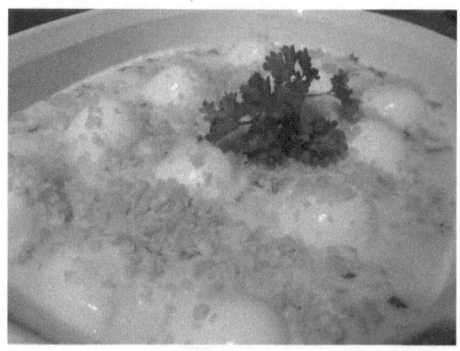

Taking the subject one level higher, it's time to start introducing egg dishes. Remember that we are trying to persuade people that do not like the taste of eggs to still include them in their diet. Cheating the taste a bit is not a great crime in the big picture of good health.

Ingredients

- 2 boiled potatoes, sliced
- 4 eggs
- 6 tablespoons of milk
- 6 tablespoons of sour cream
- 1 tablespoon flour

Method

2. Hard cook the eggs and slice them. Take a baking dish, butter it and layer the eggs and the potatoes.

3. Season with nutmeg, salt and pepper to taste. Whisk the milk, the sour cream and the flour over the layers.

4. Top with breadcrumbs. Cook at 350ºF for 25 minutes.

Potatoes

This recipe is a good choice to feed children who do not seem to be able to eat any food without potatoes. Many parents feel that eating potatoes that much is not good. On the contrary, a medium size potato contains high fiber, vitamins A, C, D, E, K, the entire complex of vitamin B, choline and betaine.

Therefore, it's not just nutritious. It's another superfood. So, with this dish, you are actually feeding your children (and yourself) with enough protection against many ailments, heart conditions, disorders and a multitude of other medical conditions that would have cost you a rather steep amount of money to the doctors and hospitals, if and when such time ever came.

163. Biscuit Sandwich

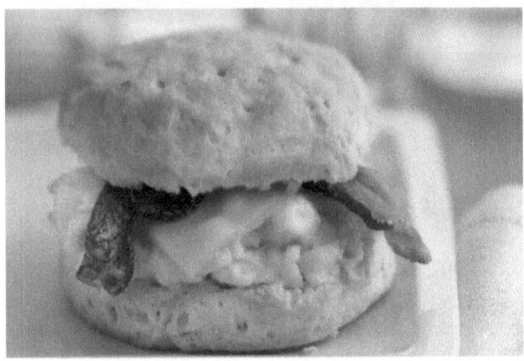

This is supposed to be a children party special, but just by reading about it, most adults would want to at least try it. It combines quite a few tasty things and is nutritious too.

Ingredients

- 2 eggs
- 1 tablespoon chopped chives
- Cheddar
- Cooked sausage patty

Method

1. Scramble the eggs (everyone knows how to do that) adding the chives. Take a biscuit and split it in two halves.

2. Take the first half melt a slice of cheddar, add the sausage patty and the eggs and top with the other half.

Tips/Notes

This is a CHILDREN's PARTY SPECIAL. Please leave some for the children (it is guaranteed that once you taste this, you will not stop eating it).

164. Migas

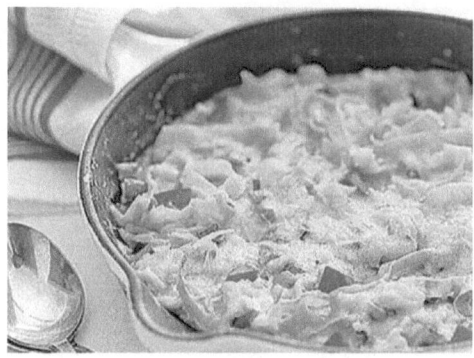

Time to start speaking a bit of Spanish. You've been speaking burritos and tortillas anyway. Time to speak migas as well. Well, speaking may be a bit of an overstatement. Probably after having this dish you'll be speechless.

Ingredients

- 4 tortillas
- 5 eggs
- Grated cheddar
- ½ cup sliced onion
- Roasted poblano peppers
- Vegetable oil
- Salsa
- Cilantro

Method

1. Make sure that the tortillas are thinly sliced and use the vegetable oil to sauté for 5 minutes in a skillet with the onion and the peppers.

2. Beat the eggs and introduce them to the skillet. Stir until the eggs are set. Top with the cheddar and the rest of the ingredients.

Tips/Notes

Vegetable oil, eggs and cheese. This combination is recommended in almost every diet that is suggested by dieticians and nutritionists worldwide. Why? Because it has all the necessary ingredients to make it a dish to control your weight and get protection from bacteria and other harmful agents.

165. Greek Family Omelet

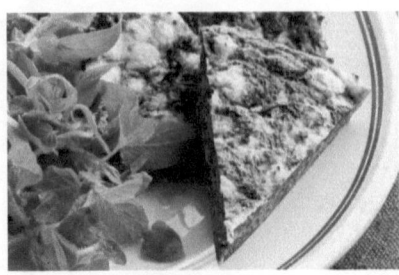

Spinach, asparagus, fruit and other omelets have been a dietary staple for decades. Time to discuss a piece of the Mediterranean diet. Since we are learning to speak multiple languages here, it seems like a very good idea.

Ingredients

- 8 eggs (or 2 for each member of the family)
- Olive oil
- 2 tablespoons of milk
- Diced ham
- Gruyere or feta cheese
- Sliced potatoes
- Tomato paste

Method

1. Cut the potatoes to French fry size and put in a frying pan and start frying with olive oil. Take the eggs and beat them in a separate bowl. Season with salt and pepper to taste.

2. If you use gruyere make sure it's well grated. If you use feta make sure it's cut to small cubes. Introduce the cheese to the bowl with the eggs and mix very well. Then introduce the tomato paste and the diced ham and keep mixing until the mixture is well-balanced.

3. About 5 minutes before the potatoes are ready, pour the mix evenly into the frying pan. Let the bottom set but not brown.

4. The traditional Greek way requires to take another frying pan, put it on top and with an abrupt and very fast move turn the omelet upside down and cook the other side too. If you cannot do that, fold the omelet like a letter.

Tips/Notes

In the other recipes, we discussed about putting one or two superfoods together. This one has four. It is strongly recommended that you do not mix this dish with other ones. An overload of nutrients may be just as dangerous as a diet that lacks them.

166. The Tri-Country Special

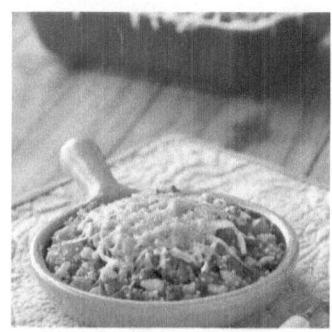

The recipe is also known as the "eggs benedict", but since we got into the habit of learning new languages, let's continue. This dish could be a very nice serving in fast food joints, if they weren't so set in serving MSG with something called food…

Ingredients

- Eggs (2 per person to be served)
- Egg yolk
- ¼ cup mayonnaise
- 1 teaspoon lemon juice
- 2 tablespoons melted butter

Method

1. The first foreign word: the Hollandaise. Take the mayo, the lemon juice, salt and pepper and puree the egg yolk in a bowl. Pulse in the butter (melted first). Make a bain marie with the bowl inside another one with simmering water and whisk until the mixture is thick.

2. Make poached eggs. Take some English muffins (OK, this may not be a foreign word), place some fried Canadian bacon on top (the third country involved), the poached eggs and cover with the Hollandaise.

Tips/Notes

The bain marie is a type of double boiler (for the uninitiated). A double boiler cannot be used in this case. It is a usual practice when you want to cook something without it getting in direct contact with the heating element or the water.

167. Eggs in Purgatory

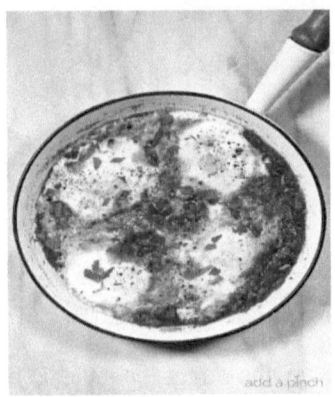

The title doesn't sound right until you take a look at the ingredients and see how easy it is to make. It could make for a very nice side dish, or a very nutritious breakfast on its own.

Ingredients

- Marinara sauce
- 6 eggs
- Parmesan

Method

1. Take a small baking dish and pour in the sauce until it is half full.

2. Crack the eggs and throw them in. Back for 10 to 12 minutes at 350°F. Whisk parmesan on top.

Tips/Notes

This is a very unique taste. And very Italian. I.e. the journey around the world continues.

168. Moroccan Eggs

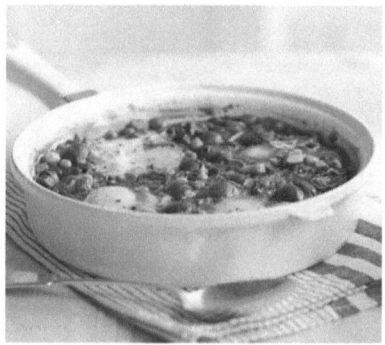

This is another style of Mediterranean diet. Still with olive oil but with enough spice to make your nostrils flame out. (No, this is not a Game of Thrones dragon primer...)

Ingredients

- 6 eggs
- 1 cup chickpeas
- Marinara sauce
- Paprika
- Ground cumin

Method

1. Take an ovenproof skillet and toast with some olive oil the chickpeas, cumin and paprika.

2. Fill the skillet with marinara sauce. Take the eggs and crack them in. Bake at 350°F for 10 to 12 minutes or until the egg whites are firm.

Tips/Notes

People all over the world have been using eggs in their cooking recognizing their great value. Each different kind of people has its own recipes and its own procedures on making very tasty dishes that can stand out.

If you want to have an informed opinion about eggs, you simply must taste them all. You may become bored, but you will probably be the healthiest person on earth. And that should count for something.

169. Nicoise Deviled Eggs

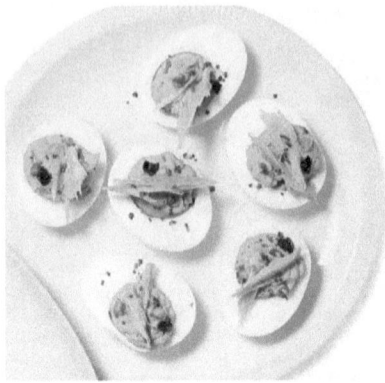

Time to go to Cyprus and Nicosia. It is also time to begin introducing more anti-oxidants and omega 3 fatty acids to the equation of the necessary nutrients to the human body.

Ingredients

- Eggs (2 per person to be served)
- 3 tablespoons olive oil
- Tuna
- Sliced olives
- Tomatoes

Method

1. Hard cook the eggs, cut in halves and take out the yolks.

2. Take a bowl and mash the olive oil, a can of tuna, some chopped parsley and some lemon juice.

3. Scoop the mash into the egg whites and top with the tomatoes and the olives.

Tips/Notes

This is one of the fastest recipes available. It can be ready for breakfast within 7 minutes, 8 tops. This will give you no more excuses to skip breakfast because you just woke up and there is no time to prepare a proper breakfast before you go to work, or sent the kids to school.

Breakfast is always the most important meal of the day. Ask any doctor you like and they will tell you the same thing. And it is one of the most important mistakes made in the western diet.

170. Ham Frittata

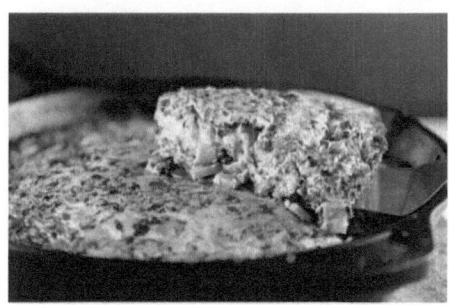

The previous recipe was a fast one. This is a slow one. However, it is also one of the tastier ones that you will find. It does have a lot of ingredients but from all accounts, it will be well worth the effort to cook it and then enjoy it. Slowly please…

Ingredients

- 8 eggs
- 3 ounces diced ham
- ½ cup milk
- 1 cup sliced asparagus
- ¾ cup shredded pecorino

Method

1. Beat the eggs, pecorino, milk with as much salt and pepper as you want. Sauté the asparagus and the ham in a skillet with olive oil.

2. Add the egg mixture and cook until the bottom sets. Bake for 25 minutes at 325°F.

Asparagus

The body does not need only amino acids, vitamins, proteins, carbs and fat. It also needs minerals like copper, manganese, phosphorus, potassium, zinc and iron. You will not easily find another food that contains as many minerals as asparagus.

In the usual manner of the superfoods, it also contains vitamins C, E, B2, B6 and K, fiber, niacin and pantothenic acid. If this all sound Greek or Chinese to you, your doctor will gladly let you know what these are all about.

171. Swiss Chard and Cheddar Quiche

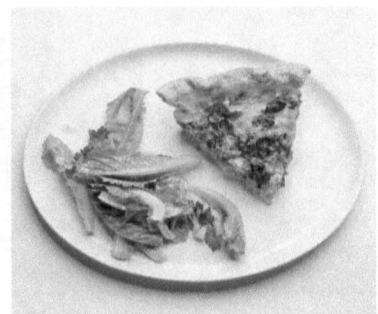

Time to take the recipes one step further. The following dish requires 15 minutes preparation and a total of an hour to cook. It is a dish very rich in calcium and properly balanced in reference to carbohydrates, fat and protein.

Ingredients

- 3 tablespoons of olive oil
- 1 tablespoon vinegar from red wine
- 1 chopped onion
- 3 eggs
- 1 9-inch prebaked piecrust
- ¾ cup half-and-half
- Kosher salt and pepper
- ½ cup of grated cheddar
- 4 cups lettuce
- 1 bunch chopped Swiss chard

Method

1. Preheat your oven to 350°F. Take a large skillet, heat one of the tablespoons of the olive oil in medium heat and add the onion and the chard. Cook for 3 to 4 minutes.

2. Take a bowl and beat the eggs with the half-and-half. Season with salt and pepper. Add the chard and the cheddar and mix. Pour onto the piecrust and bake for 40 to 45 minutes or until it sets.

3. Waiting for the baking process to be completed, use another medium bowl to mix the lettuce, the vinegar and the rest of the oil to prepare a green salad. Season with salt and pepper. Serve when it's ready in a dish with the salad on the side.

Tips/Notes

This dish contains 10 grams of saturated fat, 226 calories, 133 mg cholesterol, 813 mg of sodium, 9 grams of protein, 23 grams of carbohydrate, 3 grams of sugar, 152 mg of calcium, 2 mg of iron and 1-gram fiber.

If you are ever on a diet counting the intake, these numbers will be very useful to you.

172. Friseé with Bacon and Soft Cooked Eggs

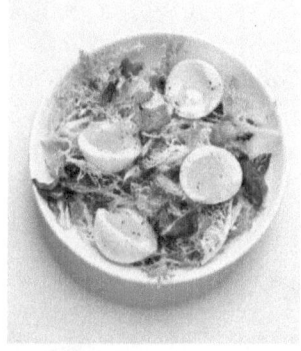

Time for dinner. All doctors will tell you that dinner should be a light meal and that it should be consumed quite some time before going to bed. Therefore, it has to be a dish that will not allow you to go sit on the couch and start dipping on snacks.

Spending 25 minutes on this dish will make it so.

Ingredients

- 8 eggs
- 3 tablespoons vinegar from red wine
- 4 cups torn friseé
- 4 slices of bacon
- 1 tablespoon of olive oil
- 4 cups of torn radicchio

Method

1. Pour some water in a medium saucepan and bring it to boil. Add the eggs very gently and boil for 6 minutes. Afterwards, rinse the eggs under cold water and peel them.

2. Cook the bacon in medium heat in a large skillet for 7 to 9 minutes or until it is crisp. Afterwards remove it, crumble it and set it aside. Add olive oil and vinegar to the bacon drippings and stir.

3. Gate a medium bowl and put in the radicchio, the friseé and the warm dressing. Toss to mix. Put the eggs and the bacon pieces on top and serve, seasoning with pepper.

Tips/Note

The ingredients refer to dinner for at least 4 people. Please leave some for the others sharing your dinner, or leave some of it for tomorrow evening as well. The temptation to eat it all at once may be too much, but you should restrain yourself.

173. Egg Pizza

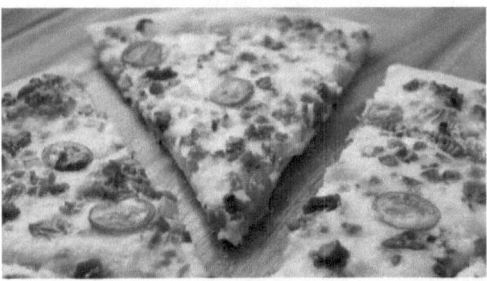

Who said that pizza had to be fattening, full of MSG, gluten and in the end bad for your health? Time to change your mind over this and definitely add pizza to your evening meals. Because there is such a thing as a healthy pizza.

Ingredients

For the dough

- ½ cup warm water
- 2 teaspoons olive oil
- ½ teaspoon salt

- About 150 grams of bread flour
- 1 teaspoon of active dry yeast

For the topping

- 3 tablespoons of olive oil
- 2 dried pepperoncini
- Fresh grated mozzarella
- 2 to 3 large eggs
- 5 garlic cloves

Method

1. Take a bowl put the water and sprinkle the yeast. Whisk until the yeast is dissolved. Cover the bowl and put it in a warm place for 5 minutes. Add the olive oil, salt and half the quantity of bread flour. Use a wooden spoon and stir for 5 minutes to form the wet dough.

2. Spread the rest of the flour on your work bench and place the wet dough on top. Start kneading and keep it up for 8 minutes or until the dough is sticky.

3. Get a large bowl and coat the sides with olive oil. Put the dough in, in the form of a ball. Roll it around to get coated in the olive oil. Cover the bowl with a towel (damp) and put in a warm place for an hour to rise.

4. Preheat the oven to 450°F and place a rack at the lower third. Peel the garlic cloves and mash them. Take 3 of them and mix them with the olive oil. Set aside.

5. Take a pizza peel or a baking pan and spread cornmeal. Push the dough to make a small round. Cover the pan and set aside for 20 minutes.

6. Use this time to take a saucepan heat some olive oil and crush the pepperoncino. Introduce the remaining garlic cloves into the oil with the pepperoncino and sauté for a minute. Add the tomato paste and loosen it with 1-2 tablespoons of water. Stir to mix. Take the saucepan out of the stovetop and set it aside.

7. Uncover the dough, press to form its final shape and spread the sauce, cheeses and two cracked eggs. Put it on a baking sheet and bake for 12 minutes at the lower third of the oven. Should you have a pizza

stone available, transfer the pizza to the stone after 8 minutes of cooking.

8. Bake until the crust is golden, take out and brush the exposed crust with the garlic oil right away.

Tips/Notes

There is such a thing as a healthy pizza, but no one said that it would be a snap to cook it. But as the saying goes, nothing that is worth doing is ever easy. It's time to think pretty hard if you prefer the pizza parlors and their MSG and gluten over a nice home made one.

By the way, you could also experiment a bit on this recipe and add a few materials like bacon and ham or mushrooms. Just some tweaking from your part and it will taste much better than what you will get from a pizza parlor.

174. Deconstructed Croque Madame

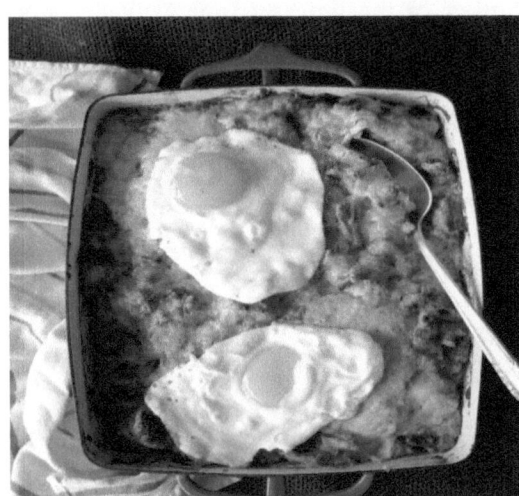

For the last recipe, we have reserved the child of a casserole and a grilled cheese sandwich. For those immersed in cooking a Croque Madame is a Croque Monsieur with an egg on top. For the uninitiated, it's all French. So, let's make it simple.

Ingredients

- 2 to 3 eggs
- A day-old brioche loaf 5 cups worth, cut in cubes

- 1¾ cups of cooked diced ham
- ¾ cups of milk
- 3 tablespoons of flour
- ¾ cup grated parmesan
- 1½ cups of grated gruyere
- 2 cups of half and half
- 1 tablespoon of canola oil
- 3 tablespoons butter

Method

1. Take a medium casserole dish, put the cubed bread inside, pour the milk and set aside. In a medium saucepan cook the ham over medium to high heat until it gets a golden-brown color. Set it aside too.

2. Preheat the oven to 400°F. You will need another medium saucepan to melt the butter in, add the flour and whisk until the mix is smooth. Add half and half and whisk until it's brought to a low boil. Allow a minute or two to thicken.

3. Add the cheeses and stir until the mix is smooth. Remove from heat and season with salt pepper and nutmeg. Place the ham on top of the bread and pour ¾ of the cheese mixture. Stir to mix thoroughly. Taste what you did and if necessary use the rest of the cheese mixture.

4. Bake for 10 to 15 minutes until it's brown on top. Meanwhile take a medium saucepan and heat a tablespoon of oil until it's hot, in medium to high heat. Add the eggs gently and cook until the white is done but the yolk is still intact. This should take about three minutes.

5. Take the casserole out of the oven, top with the eggs and serve immediately

Tips/Notes

The language lesson ended with a French touch. It's not expected that you became fluent with all the languages we presented, but with some practice, you will learn to speak all of them.

Conclusion

Well, that's it! Good nutrition is the start point of your journey towards reducing your any chances of developing a health problem. Making these very tasty and healthy recipes at home is also a great way of controlling health problems such as blood pressure, cholesterol levels and diabetes just to name a few.

The aim of creating these recipes is to help you prepare meals that are not only tasty but also add a significant amount of nutritional value for you. Most importantly, you are what you eat and it's time to get back control in your life. Learn to adapt to change, particularly with your food attitude for an opportunity to change your life!

Final Words

I would like to thank you for downloading my book and I hope I have been able to help you and educate you about something new.

If you have enjoyed this book and would like to share your positive thoughts, could you please take 30 seconds of your time to go back and give me a review on my Amazon book page!

I greatly appreciate seeing these reviews because it helps me share my hard work!

Again, thank you and I wish you all the best with your weight loss journey!

Disclaimer

This book and related site provides recipe and food advice in an informative and educational manner only, with information that is general in nature and that is not specific to you, the reader. The contents of this book and related site are intended to assist you and other readers in your personal efforts. Consult your physician or nutritionist regarding the applicability of any information provided in our information to you.

Nothing in this book should be construed as personal advice or diagnosis, and must not be used in this manner. The information provided about conditions is general in nature. This information does not cover all possible uses, actions, precautions, side-effects, or interactions of medicines, or medical procedures. The information in this site should not be considered as complete and does not cover all diseases, ailments, physical conditions, or their treatment.

No Warranties: The authors and publishers don't guarantee or warrant the quality, accuracy, completeness, timeliness, appropriateness or suitability of the information in this book, or of any product or services referenced by this site.

The information in this site is provided on an "as is" basis and the authors and publishers make no representations or warranties of any kind with respect to this information. This site may contain inaccuracies, typographical errors, or other errors.

Liability Disclaimer: The publishers, authors, and other parties involved in the creation, production, provision of information, or delivery of this site specifically disclaim any responsibility, and shall not be held liable for any damages, claims, injuries, losses, liabilities, costs, or obligations including any direct, indirect, special, incidental, or consequences damages (collectively known as "Damages") whatsoever and howsoever caused, arising out of, or in connection with the use or misuse of the site and the information contained within it, whether such Damages arise in contract, tort, negligence, equity, statute law, or by way of other legal theory.

www.ingramcontent.com/pod-product-compliance
Lightning Source LLC
Chambersburg PA
CBHW031110080526
44587CB00011B/909